I0437051

The Poisoning of Americans

The Poisoning of Americans

A Tale of Congress, the FDA, the Agricultural Department, and Chemical and Pharmaceutical Companies and How They Work Together to Reduce the Health and Life Span of Americans

JACOB SILVER, PhD

iUniverse, Inc.
Bloomington

The Poisoning of Americans
A Tale of Congress, the FDA, the Agricultural Department, and
Chemical and Pharmaceutical Companies and How They Work
Together to Reduce the Health and Life Span of Americans

Copyright © 2012 by Jacob Silver, PhD

All rights reserved. No part of this book may be used or reproduced by any means,
graphic, electronic, or mechanical, including photocopying, recording, taping or by any
information storage retrieval system without the written permission of the publisher
except in the case of brief quotations embodied in critical articles and reviews.

Neither the author of the publisher shall be liable for any loss or damage allegedly arising
as a consequence of your use or application of any information contained in this book.

iUniverse books may be ordered through booksellers or by contacting:

iUniverse
1663 Liberty Drive
Bloomington, IN 47403
www.iuniverse.com
1-800-Authors (1-800-288-4677)

Because of the dynamic nature of the Internet, any web addresses or links contained in this book may
have changed since publication and may no longer be valid. The views expressed in this work are
solely those of the author and do not necessarily reflect the views of the publisher, and the publisher
hereby disclaims any responsibility for them.

Any people depicted in stock imagery provided by Thinkstock are models,
and such images are being used for illustrative purposes only.

Certain stock imagery © Thinkstock.

ISBN: 978-1-4759-4196-8 (sc)
ISBN: 978-1-4759-4197-5 (hc)
ISBN: 978-1-4759-5306-0 (e)

Library of Congress Control Number: 2012914314

Printed in the United States of America

iUniverse rev. date: 8/28/2012

Contents

Introduction

THAT ARSENIC HAS BEEN added to chicken feed[1] in chicken factory farms, and ammonia is added to ground beef of factory farms[2] demonstrates the aptness of the title of this book. And it is not just arsenic. Factory farm chickens are also fed caffeine, the active ingredients of Tylenol and Benadryl, and some banned antibiotics.[3] If this sounds strange to the reader, and it should, one must understand the circumstances behind such administrations.

First of all, chickens are fairly self-contained animals. In my youth, we raised chickens, for eggs, but we also ate some of them. These chickens roamed around on our little farm, scratching the dirt, and pecking what they found. They were up a dawn. They did not need caffeine. They did get nervous sometimes. Dogs got too close. A hawk might have flown overhead. But these incidents passed. It would never have occurred to us to administer drugs or caffeine to these chickens. But these were free range chickens, even before that phrase became current. The chickens referred to in the first paragraph are not free range chickens, they are factory farm chickens. And that gets to the basis of it. We will discuss chicken factory farms in Chapter 4. But for now two points are relevant.

The first point is that in chicken factory farms, 4 to 11 hens are put into a cage which is two foot wide and two foot long, and barely two foot

---

1   Roxarsone, and FDA approved drug for chickens, is arsenic based. Then, in June 2011 the FDA ordered Pfizer, the parent company of its manufacture, to discontinue selling the drug.

2   The New York Times, December 31, 2009.

3   Nicholas D. Kristof, the New York Times, April 5, 2012.

high. They cannot spread their wings. Their "purpose" is to lay eggs. And they do so on a forward slanting floor, which rolls the egg out of the cage. Otherwise the eggs would be trampled. There is a line of these cages. And there is a line of cages directly above. Which means that excrement passes through to the chickens below. This is where supermarket "fresh eggs" come from. So, given this unusual and inhumane system, chickens are given mood stabilizers and stimulants to encourage them to lay. But these chickens cannot scratch. They cannot eat larvae or insects. They cannot run, or fly to a low branch. They cannot develop the normal musculature of a normal chicken. They cannot be considered healthy.

And their diet is a mixture, mostly corn. It provides these chickens with no omega 3 oils. More on this later. And the companies which control these factory farms have no hesitation to sell their product as "fresh eggs."

With regard to ammonia added to ground beef, there is an explanation. Ground beef is made from particular muscle meat, to which is added the fat trimmings which were formally sold to the pet food industry, or for tallow manufacture. Well, these fat trimmings are probably contaminated with e-coli 0157:H7. This is not the normal type of e-coli in cattle. In grass fed cattle the e-coli is PH neutral. But in the corn fed cattle of feed lots, the e-coli is a mutation referred to as e-coli 0157:H7. This is an acid resistant e-coli, and if consumed by humans, can be fatal. So, it is reasonable that factory farms would apply ammonia to their ground beef to kill the e-coli 0157:H7. What is not reasonable is that they have forced cattle to develop e-coli 0157:H7 by feeding them corn. And it is unconscionable that they gather up the fat trimmings to include in their ground beef, and to *pasteurize* this mixture by the addition of ammonia.

Of course things are a bit more complicated. With respect to ammonia, it comes in diluted and concentrated forms. A diluted form, with a PH of 6, has no adverse effects if ingested. A PH of 6 is as acidic as milk or rainwater. But the United States Department of Agriculture (USDA), sympathetic with the beef industry, approved the use of ammonia with a PH as high as 10. This is caustic, and is lethal to e-coli 0157:H7. It may well be lethal to all bacteria, which means that it could cause havoc among the intestinal bacteria of a person eating such a hamburger.

With respect to arsenic, it comes in two types of compounds. "Organic arsenic," which is present naturally in the earth and in foods is not readily toxic, and "inorganic arsenic. On average, most people have about 10-20 mg of organic arsenic in their bodies. It is known that this level causes no problems in the human body. Higher levels may lead to problems. But intake is usually very low, and much of it is eliminated in the feces and some in the urine. And the Pfizer drug, Roxarsone, contains organic arsenic, but at a higher level than what is usually consumed. This drug is administered to kill parasites, particularly coccidiosis. This is a disease of factory farm chickens. The chickens of my youth, and the chickens of farms which allow the chickens to roam free range, do not encounter such diseases. But, if we have factory farms, we have to administer drugs which deal with the disease generation which these factory farms foster. And does the inclusion of Roxarsone in chicken feed lead to any problems? Well, yes it does. Whenever you disturb the natural equilibrium, you are going to cause problems. The Food and Drug Administration (FDA) found that Roxarsone produced inorganic arsenic, a known carcinogen, in the livers of chickens administered that drug.[4] It was further found that the manure of chickens fed Roxarsone, converted the arsenic to inorganic arsenic.[5] Farmers spread this manure over their land. Now the good news: Pfizer announced that it will discontinue the sales of Roxarsone in the United States. Of course it will continue to sell Roxarsone overseas where it is allowed. They are not going to lose out on profit, are they?

To understand all of these matters properly, and to grasp the magnitude of the problem, we should start first with the fundamentals.

---

4   Http://www.fda.gov/AnimalVeterinary/Safety   Health/Product   Safety Information

5   Http://www.worldpoultry.net/news/roxarsone-in-chicken-feed-causes risks-to-humans

1 - Fundamentals

HUMANS AND HUMAN FOOD

HUMANS SHARE ABOUT 98.5% of our genes with the Bonobo, otherwise known as the Pigmy Chimpanzee. That is closer than the genetic relationship we have with any other species. Minimally that implies that we share a common ancestor with the Bonobo. Our main differences are our brain and our neotenic[6] body shape. But our organs, including our digestive system, are practically identical, implying that the joint evolution that brought us here equipped us for similar diets.

What does the Bonobo eat?

This primate is mainly frugivorous, but supplements its diet with leaves and sometimes small vertebrates (such as flying squirrels and infant duikers) and invertebrates.[7]

So, our nearest evolutionary relative eats mainly a vegetarian diet, with an admixture of some meat. Our mutual digestive system is quite suited to such a diet. We have a slightly acidic stomach which can break down meat, provided it is surrounded with vegetable matter. Our digestive system is

---

6   Neoteny refers to speciation wherein the new individual(s) retain infant physical characteristics even as they grow to adulthood. Humans, emerging from the ape line of primates, have short arms, a hairless body, and a relatively flat face, the characteristics of an infant Bonobo. But we could not have evolved from Bonobos; the relation we have with Bonobos is a probable common ancestor.

7   http://en.wikipedia.org/wiki/Bonobo - 'Duikers' are a small antelope.

twelve times the length of our body[8], a long digestive tract suited to break down fruits, vegetables, grains, and nuts. We no longer have a functioning appendix[9], which Bonobos still do have. Thus, the only safe way for us to digest meat, particularly a substantial clump of meat, is to first break it down by heating, broiling, grilling, baking, or frying. But our long digestive system tells us that our body does not expect to have to digest a large quantity of meat; it is designed for fruits, nuts, grains, and vegetables.

Persons who enjoy eating meat have occasionally compared humans with carnivores. This, of course, is biological nonsense. But it may be instructive to make a brief comparison of the diets and digestive systems of carnivores, as compared to humans. First of all, using the Grey Wolf as an example, carnivores have a very acidic stomach, containing hydrochloric acid, as does the stomach of human, but wolves' stomach contains 20 times the acidity of human stomachs.[10] And the digestive tract of carnivores is much shorter than that of humans, about three times the length of their bodies. This is well suited to the normal diet of carnivores, which is almost the exclusive consumption of raw meat. The only exception is their consumption of the vegetable contents of the digestive tracts of their prey. So, with a diet which is 98% or 99% raw meat, it is essential that it be processed quickly, and expelled quickly, before the meat spoils. Thus, the digestive system and diet of carnivores is very unlike that of humans. And to the degree that humans may try to eat in the manner of carnivores, making the single concession of having their largely meat diet cooked, the consequences are the consumption of saturated fat, higher cholesterol, and heart disease. Heart disease, high blood pressure, and high cholesterol are not natural or unavoidable. They are largely attributable to diet.

CATTLE

CATTLE WERE DOMESTICATED ABOUT seven thousand years ago, during the early neolithic period, probably in what is now northern Greece.[11] Cattle

---

8   Lyman, Howard F. MAD COWBOY, (Simon & Schuster, New York), pp. 182-183

9   The human appendix is not involved in direct digestion, but it does harbor intestinal bacteria, which can emerge and can compensate the other intestinal bacteria were they to become reduced.

10   *Idem.*

11   Harper, Douglas (2001). Cattle. Online Etymological Dictionary. Retrieved on 2007-06-13.

are bovine animals, and the word 'cattle' derives from the Latin *caput,* meaning head, and from the middle English *chattel,* meaning a unit of personal property. The people originally domesticating cattle undoubtedly noticed that these animals subsist on grasses, and could be maintained on land too poor to grow other crops. So, while the best land produced legumes, grains, and vegetables, the sparse grasslands could now produce milk and/or meat and leather. But right from the beginning, cattle were valuable possessions, and the slaughter of cattle for meat and leather was not a frequent thing. People did not eat meat frequently. They subsisted mostly on fruits, nuts, grains, legumes, and vegetables.

So, what are cattle, evolutionarily and taxonomically? First they are mammals, just as humans are. Their sub-order is Ruminantia, including grazing animals which chew their cud. Their family is Bovidae, and that is made up of cattle, goats, sheep, and antelope, and a few others. All of these members of the family Bovidae are grass eaters. They have long and complex digestive systems, with four compartments, otherwise known as four 'stomachs' or one stomach with four chambers. The first compartment is called the rumen. The rumen contains bacteria which break down the cellulose of the grass.[12] This is a difficult process; thus, Bovidae regurgitate the contents of the rumen and continue to chew them. This is 'chewing the cud.' This is swallowed again, and the bacteria work further on the process of breaking it down. Then it progresses to the other compartments, and then through the digestive tract. Because the breakdown, to extract needed nutrients, involves fermentation, the digestive system of ruminants, those who 'chew the cud,' is PH neutral.

This circumstance, of Bovidae not having an acidic digestive system, allowed lions, tigers, and wolves to eat these animals without aggravating their already highly acidic digestive systems. When humans eat antelope or cattle, which are grass fed, they also do not get acidic poisoning. For thousands of years humans have eaten cattle with no danger of acidic poisoning.

A common constituent in mammalian digestive systems is the bacterium Escherichia coli, also known as E coli. Cattle have Escherichia coli, as do humans. It is a normal part of our digestive system's bacterial colony. But in recent years there has been a concern, and a number of victims, of ' E-coli poisoning.' Reference is the E-coli emanating from slaughtered cattle. Now, it must be understood that E-coli are bacteria, and are very small. And traditionally, when cattle were slaughtered and

---

12   http://en.wikipedia.org/wiki/Cattle

butchered, some of the E-coli got out, and on and in the muscle or meat of the animal, which people consume. But, as I have stated in the preceding paragraph, there is no danger of poisoning from the eating of E-coli from grass fed cattle. But most of the cattle which are slaughtered and butchered in the United States today are not grass fed. They are confined in feed lots, and fed corn, along with antibacterial drugs, animal protein, and ground up plastic. These will be discussed below. But now it should be understood that the feeding of corn to cattle, a member of Bovidae, is unnatural. The digestive system of cattle is not structured to digest corn. The bacterial colony within the rumen cannot process corn. But if the only food they receive is corn, and normal E-coli cannot process it, a reversion occurs to an earlier type of E-coli, referred to as Escherichia coli 0157:H7. This is an acidic bacterium, and it is poisonous to consume.

BACTERIA

BACTERIA ARE ALL ABOUT us. In terms of distribution and biomass, bacteria are the dominant life form on Earth. And when considering multi-celled animals, bacteria are an integral part of just about all of them. Certainly for people and cattle, the bacteria in our gut are an integral part of our system.[13] Consider an adult human. She has about 100 billion cells of her own, with her own DNA. She also has about one trillion bacteria in her gut, and elsewhere in the body. She, as is true for all humans, and probably all large animals, has ten times more bacterial cells in her body than her own cells. This is a sobering thought. What, then, are people? We are not simple individuals. We are a commensal-life form, encompassing many different lives. And, of course, these bacteria are friendly, in the sense that your arm is friendly. They are an essential part of our system. They participate in the digestion of our food.

Beyond the symbiotic bacteria in our intestines, scientists are discovering symbiotic bacteria throughout our skin.[14] A recent finding is that there are several million bacteria inhabiting the inner elbow of every human.[15] These are symbiotic, they receive shelter and nourishment in

---

13   http://en.wikipedia.org/wiki/Bacteria

14   Gorman, James. "Aliens Inside Us: A (Mostly Friendly) Bacterial Nation," The New York Times, (Science Section), April 1, 2003.

15   15Wade, Nicholas. "Bacteria Thrive in Inner Elbow; No Harm Done," The New York Times, (Science Section), May 23, 2008.

exchange for moisturizing our elbows by processing the raw fats. They are also called commensal bacteria. They are part of our system. When a person says "I," she means all of her own cells plus all of her symbiotic bacterial colonies. It is one system.

Other friendly bacteria include those which make cheese or yogurt.[16] Gardeners and farmers who grow beans, inoculate their bean seeds with bacteria which fix nitrogen from the air, and bacteria are the essential elements in sewerage treatment plants, where they break down sewerage to harmless components. These are only the most conspicuous bacteria that people are acquainted with and employ.

There are hostile bacteria, bacteria whose functioning in our lungs or gut would make us ill. There are bacteria which are lethal to people. But, for the most part, bacteria in the air, on the ground, and on and in the food we eat are, mostly, harmless, neutral. There is constant interaction with hostile bacteria, but we are armed with antibodies, which destroy those bacteria before they get a chance to do any mischief. It is the nature of life, and of human life, to be in a constant state of challenge. We are always experiencing new bacteria, and we build, in response, new antibodies.

Finally, there are pathogenic bacteria which are associated with serious illnesses. Some of the most common of these have names we recognize: Anthrax, Tuberculosis, and Cholera. Anthrax[17] enters to lungs and skin of a human who comes in contact with an infected animal or other human. It migrates to the lungs and lymph glands. It is often fatal. Cholera[18] enters the gastro-intestinal system from the ingestion of contaminated food or water. Tuberculosis, caused by the bacterium Mycobacterium tuberculosis[19], generally enters a person's lungs by inhalation. But 25% of all cases involve the attack of the person's neural system, or lymph system, or circulatory system, or the genitourinary system. About 1.6 million deaths occur annually from tuberculosis, primarily in developing countries.

To counter these, and other, pathogenic bacteria, antibiotic drugs have been developed. The name was chosen to indicate that the original intent was to have a pharmaceutical agent to kill hostile fungi as well as bacteria.

---

16   Among the bacteria in yogurt, lactobacillus acidophilus and lactobacillus casei, are normally resident in the human body.

17   http://en.wikipedia.org/wiki/Anthrax

18   http://en.wikipedia.org/wiki/Cholera

19   http://en.wikipedia.org/wiki/Tuberculosis

However, the current roster of antibiotics are anti-bacterial only. Antibiotics work, generally, by attacking the cell wall. Of all the cells operating in the human system, only bacteria have cell walls. Humans, and animals, have cell membranes, which are chemically different. The pathogenic bacteria have cell walls, but the commensal bacteria, which are part of our intestinal system, also have cell walls. Antibiotic drugs are, therefore, a threat to us. Harm to the human system can be mitigated with targeting the area of the antibiotic as well as the type of antibiotic. Our lungs are, obviously, aerobic. Our digestive tract is anaerobic. Thus, all of our beneficial bacteria in our large intestine are anaerobic. If an antibiotic is effective against tuberculosis or another lung affecting bacterium, it does not affect processes in our digestive tract.[20] However if an antibiotic is used against a pathogen in our digestive tract, harm can be avoided, or limited, if it is restricted to the stomach, where Heliobacter pylori usually resides, or its effectiveness is restricted to the particular pathogen. Another way of saying this is whether the antibiotic is narrow or broad spectrum. Broad spectrum antibiotics administered in the digestive tract usually also kill many commensal bacteria. The immediate symptoms of this are abdominal distress and diarrhea. Usually, some of the beneficial bacteria survive, and, in a few days, they can reconstitute their ranks. If a particularly large dose of a broad spectrum antibiotic were administered, all of the symbiotic bacteria could be killed. The consequence would continuing severe abdominal stress and diarrhea, and a deficiency in vitamin K. There would also be a growing deficiency in amino acids and nutrients normally processed by the intestinal bacteria. Until such bacteria are replaced, life for that person would not be normal.

So, remembering who we are, that we are bacterial colonies as well as own cells, we should not be cavalier or mindlessly careless about the use of antibiotics in our system. And when they have to be used, they should be very carefully targeted. The specific thing to remember is that we, all of us, are permanent walking alliances of human cells and bacterial colonies. The health of a person depends on the health of all of the members of this alliance. Certainly, we should not take poison which would hurt any part of us, because any part of us is us.

The Great Plains of the United States

We have just discussed humans, Bonobos, cattle, and bacteria, all living things. And now the subtitle says we are going to discuss a geographic

---

20   But it might affect the aerobic commensal bacteria resident in our mouth.

phenomenon. Well, the subtitles of this chapter are the topics which are relevant to our discussion of the major food production system in America. And the great plains of the United States is a major factor in this system. The Great Plains of the United States is an extensive prairie land east of the Rocky Mountains. It includes eastern Montana, western North Dakota, most of South Dakota, the eastern third of Wyoming, half of Colorado, most of Nebraska, and the western two thirds of Kansas. To the north it extends to Canada, and to the south it extends to the Rio Grande.[21]

Before Europeans came to North America, the Great Plains, except for the flood plains of rivers and the foothills of the Rockies, were totally covered in grass. This provided a habitat for very large herds of bison, a member of the cud chewing, grass eating Bovidae family of which cattle are members. Trees did not grow because the Great Plains is a semi-arid area, receiving only 20 inches or less of rain annually.[22] Such an arid area can also only support a sparse human population, and the Native American population of the Great Plains, as compared to the Native American populations around the Great Lakes and along the East Coast, was sparse indeed.

Beneath most of the Great Plains is a huge aquifer, one of the world's largest. It lies beneath 174,000 squared miles (450,000 km^2) in portions of the eight states of South Dakota, Nebraska, Wyoming, Colorado, Kansas, Oklahoma, New Mexico, and Texas.[23] This aquifer was named the Ogallala Aquifer after the name of the town, Ogallala, Kansas, where it was discovered in 1899. It has also been referred to as the Oglala Aquifer. "About 27 percent of the irrigated land in the United States overlies this aquifer system, which yields about 30 percent of the nation's water taken from the ground and used for irrigation. In addition, the aquifer system provides drinking water to 82 percent of the people who live within the aquifer boundary."[24]

The water permeated thickness of the aquifer varies from 1,000 feet (300m) to 100 feet (30m). The deepest water is in the northern plains. Generally, the water below the surface ranges from 400 feet (122m) in the north to between 100 to 200 feet (30 to 61m) in the south. "Present-day

---

21   http://en.wikipedia.org/wiki/Great_Plains

22   Trimble, Donald E. "The Geologic Story of the Great Plains." GEOLOGIC SURVEY BULLETIN 1493, United States Government Printing Office, Washington, D.C., 1980.

23   http://en.wikipedia.org/wiki/Ogallala_Aquifer

24   *Idem.*

recharge of the aquifer with fresh water occurs at a slow rate; this implies that much of the water in its pore spaces is paleowater, dating back to the last ice age."[25] The last ice age ended about 12,000 years ago.

An aquifer may be conceived as a groundwater storage reservoir in the water cycle. Aquifers renew much more slowly than does groundwater. Yet inflow to a aquifer has to also come from the surface. Outflow can be baseflow to streams. In recent years major outflow has also occurred by pumping.

> The rate at which recharge water enters the aquifer is limited by several factors. Much of the plains region is semi-arid with steady winds that hasten evaporation of surface water and precipitation. In many locations, the aquifer is overlain, in the vadose zone, with a shallow layer of caliche that is practically impermeable; this limits the amount of water able to recharge the aquifer from the land surface. However, the soil of the playa lakes is different and not lined with caliche, making these some of the few areas where the aquifer can recharge. The destruction of playas by farmers and development then decreases the available recharge area.[26]

The ' vadose zone' is the geologic zone between the surface layer and the saturated area of the aquifer. It is also, therefore, known as the unsaturated zone. " Caliche" is a hardened crust or layer of calcium carbonate. It is formed by the evaporation of water solutions of the mineral. Deserts and semi-arid areas are often covered with caliche. " Playa lakes" or areas refer to the bottoms of dry lakes. In semi-arid regions, a playa lake may be full of water during the winter or rainy season, and then soaks in and evaporates to leave a dry lake during most of the rest of the year.

So we see that the Ogallala Aquifer is a very large subterranean body of ancient water. Ancient, in part, because recharging is very slow. Maintaining a balance between inflow (charging) and outflow would mean maintaining the proper level of population and activity affordable by this semi-arid plains area. But there is no balance being maintained with the Ogallala Aquifer. Each year 420 billion cubic feet (12 billion m³) is pumped out, amounting to a total depletion, to date, of a volume equal to the annual flow of 18 Colorado Rivers. It is estimated that, at this rate of depletion, the aquifer will dry up in as early as 2033.

---

25   http://en.wikipedia.org/wiki/Ogallala_Aquifer, p. 2

26   *Idem.*

2 - Essential Fatty Acids and Health

To SURVIVE, THE HUMAN body requires the acquisition of substances from its environment. These include oxygen, water, light, a source of energy, 8 essential amino acids, 13 vitamins, 20 or 21 elements, referred to dietarily as 'minerals,' and two fatty acids.[27] These fatty acids are α-linolenic acid and linoleic acid, referred to as the omega 3 and omega 6 fatty acids, respectively.

The omega fatty acids are polyunsaturates[28] which are essential nutrients for humans. They must be obtained from food.[29] Plants can make these fatty acids, but humans cannot. These fatty acids are related to the physiological and neurological health of humans.[30]

The omega 3 fatty acid is α-Linolenic acid, or ALA or LNA (18:3). It is a polyunsaturated fatty acid which cannot be synthesized by humans. Once α-Linolenic acid is acquired, it is catalyzed into two long chain polyunsaturated fatty acids, which are:

---

27 Erasmus, Udo. Fats that Heal; Fats that Kill, Chapter 13, "Essential Nutrients," pp. 73-82.

28 Polyunsaturates are polyunsaturated fatty acids which have two or more cis (configuration isomerism) double bonds which are separated from each other by a single methylene group. The essential fatty acids are omega-3 and -6.

29 http://en.wikipedia.org/wiki/Omega-3_fatty_acid

30 http://www.unnews.com/articles/new/50-ways-to-improve-your-life and http://www.eatwild.com/healthbenefits.htm and Rose, DP & Connolly, JM "Effects of Dietary Omega-3 Fatty Acids on Human Breast Cancer Growth and Metastases in Nude Mice," in http://www.nebi.nlm.ih.gov/pubmed/8411258

eicosapentaenoic acid (EPA, 20:5), and
docosahexaenoic acid (DHA, 22:6).

The omega 6 fatty acid is Linoleic acid, or LA (18:2). Once it is acquired, the human body catalyzes three long chain fatty acids, which are:

gamma-linolenic acid (GLA, 18:3),
[from GLA] dihomo-gamma-linolenic acid (DGLA, 20:3),
and
arachidonic acid (AA, 20:4)[31]

Eicosapentaenoic acid (EPA) has been clinically demonstrated to be effective in the treatment of coronary artery disease, hypertension, diabetes, arthritis, other inflammatory and autoimmune disorders, and cancer.[32] It has also been demonstrated to be an effective treatment for depression and schizophrenia.[33] There is also strong evidence from human trials that using both eicosapentaenoic acid (EPA) and docosahexaenoic acid (DHA) together, from fish or fish oil supplements, significantly reduces blood triglyceride levels.[34] Several studies also report that the regular consumption of oily fish or fish oil, which has a high proportion of both EPA and DHA, reduces the risk of non-fatal heart attacks, fatal heart attacks, sudden death, and deaths due to any pathological cause in people with histories of heart attacks.[35]

It should be said that all fats, or fatty acids, in the human body are transported through the arteries and veins as triglycerides. This refers to the

---

31   http://en.widkipedia.org/widi/Essential_fatty_acid

32   Simopoulos, Artemis P. "Omega-3 fatty acids in wild plants, nuts and seeds," Asia Pacific Journal of Clinical Nutrition (2002) 11(S6), p. S163 and Yokoyama, M., Origasa H., Matsuzaki M., Saito Y, et alia, "Effects of Eicosapentaenoic acit on major coronary events in hypercholesterolaemic patients (JELIS): a randomized open-label, blinded endpoint analysis," found in http://www.ncbi.nlm.nih.gov/pubmed/17398303

33   Song C., and Zhao S. "Omega-3 fatty acid eicosapentaenoic acid. A new treatment for psychiatric and neurodegenerative diseases: a review of clinical investigations," in http://www.nebi.nlm.nih.gov/pubmed/17922626?ordinalpos=1 &itoo

34   Omega-3 fatty acids, fish oil, alpha-linolenic acid," in Medline Plus, in http://www.nlm.nih.gov/medlineplus/druginfo/natural/patient-fishoil

35   *Idem.*

joining of three fat molecules to a glycerin atom. The resulting structure is a triglyceride. The discussion in this chapter is of specific fats which are delivered to cells in the form of triglycerides. The cell processes treat each fat separately. The discussion here is the processing of the omega 3 and 6 fats.

Docosahexaenoic acid (DHA), from α-Linolenic acid, through oxygenation form signaling molecules, including some resolvins and the docosatrienes. Resolvins and docosatrienes are bioactive compounds which demonstrate potent anti-inflammatory and immunoregulatory actions.[36] Resolvins specifically act to reduce inflammation by inhibiting the transport of inflammatory cells to the site of an inflammation. DHA is metabolized to form docosanoids, which are a family of potent hormones. DHA is also a major fatty acid in sperm and brain phospholipids, and also especially in the retina.

Before we discuss the omega 6 fatty acid long chain derivatives, it should be understood that, as with other nutrients, omega 3 fatty acids and omega 6 fatty acids contribute constructively, positively, to physiological maintenance and integrity only by working together, in roughly equal proportions. Prior to the huge United States' corn subsidy and the emergence of factory farms, the ratio of omega 6 fatty acids to omega 3 fatty acids taken in with food was 1:1 to 4:1. This is a healthy range, and it precluded many of the adverse medical conditions and diseases which have faced Americans in recent years. The reconstructed evidence, derived from some archeological findings and from an analysis of the diet of the few current hunting and gathering populations still on Earth, indicates that the human evolutionary diet was close to an omega 6 to 3 ratio of 1:1.[37] The medical trials and studies cited above, involving the remedial effects of the administration of large doses of omega 3 fatty acids, indicates that it was a restorative treatment. The conditions treated, heart disease and schizophrenia, were omega 3 fatty acid deficiency conditions. This simply expands the meaning of the lead sentence of this paragraph, that human

---

36   Serhan CN, Gotlinger K, Hong S, Arita M. "Resolvins, docosatrienes, and neuroprotectins, novel omega-3-derived mediators, and their aspirin-triggered endogenous epimers: an overview of their protective roles in catabasis." Prostaglandins Other Lipid Mediat. 2004 Apr;73(3-4):155-72, 156

37   Simopoulos, ibid, pp 163-164, also Simopoulos, Artemis P. "The omega-6/omega-3 fatty acid ratio, genetic variation, and cardiovascular disease," Asia Pacific Journal of Clinical Nutrition (2008): 17 (S1): pp. 131-134.

health depends on the consumption of a healthy ratio range of omega 6 and omega 3 fatty acids.

Gamma-linolenic acid (GLA) is a long chain derivative of linoleic acid (LA), also known as the omega 6 fatty acid. GLA is unique among omega 6 polyunsaturated fatty acids, linoleic acid and arachidonic acid, in its potential to suppress tumor growth and metastasis. Because it has demonstrated these abilities to some, research is ongoing to establish GLA as an anticancer agent. It has also been claimed as treatment for autoimmune disorders, arthritis, eczema, and PMS.[38]

The major role of GLA in the maintenance of the human body is that it is the source of dihomo-gamma-linolenic acid (DGLA). DGLA, along with arachidonic acid (AA) and eicosapentaenoic acid (EPA), are the three sole sources of eicosanoids, which are the signaling molecules in each human cell. DGLA, through its derivatives, inhibits the pro-inflammatory signals of the derivatives of AA. Gamma-linolenic acid (GLA), through dihomo-gama-linolenic acid (DGLA) serves an anti-inflammatory role in the human body.

Arachidonic acid (AA) is the second derivative of linoleic acid (LA), and is the third major fatty acid derivative of linoleic acid. Arachidonic acid produces several eicosanoids. One is thromboxane, which is a powerful vasoconstrictor and it increases platelet aggregation. Others signal inflammation, and they contract smooth muscle, which are the bronchi and blood vessel. Thus, they promote asthma and hypertension,[39] when arachidonic acid is not counterbalanced with other, chiefly, omega 3, fatty acids.

Arachidonic acid, itself, is abundantly present in the brain, and it also is present in the phospholipids, the cell membranes, of each cell.[40] If arachidonic acid in the brain is disproportionately represented, not counterbalanced by omega 3 fatty acids, it hyperfunctions to produce

---

38 http://en.wikipedia.org/wiki/Gamma-Linolenic_acid

39 "The Arachidonic Acid Pathway," by drdoc on-line, in http://www.arthritis.co.za/arachid.html

40 http://en.wikipedia.org/wiki/Arachidonic_acid

the conditions of depression and schizophrenia.[41] If arachidonic acid in cell membranes is disproportionately represented, not counterbalanced by omega 3 fatty acids, it hyperfunctions to cause tumor growth.

An omega-6 fatty acid known as arachidonic acid turns on a gene signaling pathway that leads directly to tumor growth, according to principal investigator Millie Hushes-Fulford, Ph.D., director of the Laboratory of Cell Growth at SFVAMC (San Francisco VA Medical Center) and scientific advisor to the U.S. Under Secretary for Health for the Department of Veterans Affairs.[42]

The disproportionate distribution of arachidonic acid in the body can also cause breast cancer:

Diets rich in omega-6 polyunsaturated fatty acids stimulate the growth and metastases of transplantable mammary carcinomas in rodents, whereas fish oil-containing diets, rich in omega-3 fatty acids, suppress the growth of these mammary tumor cells.[43]

The disproportionate distribution of arachidonic acid, not counterbalanced by omega 3 fatty acids, has also been cited as causative of diabetes, arthritis, and autoimmune disorders.[44]

Arachidonic acid, and its derivative eicosanoids, are very active in the human body, and left alone, i.e., not counterbalanced with omega 3

---

41   Peet, Malcolm; Brind, Jan; Ramchand, C. N.; Shah, Sandeep; and Vankar, G. K. "Two double-blind placebo-controlled pilot studies of eicosapentaenoic acid in the treatment of schizophrenia," SCHIZOPHRENIA RESEARCH 49 (2001) pp. 243-251 and Song, c and Zhao, S. "Omega-3 fatty acid eicosapentaenoic acid. A new treatment for psychiatric and neurodegenerative diseases: a review of clinical investigations," Expert opin Investig Drugs, 2007 Oct: 16 (10): 1627-38 in http://www.ncbi.nlm.nih.gov/pubmed/17922626?ordinalpos=1&itoo

42   "Fatty acids such as those found in corn oil turn on genes that stimulate tumor growth," News-Medical.Net, at http://www.news-medical.net/print_article.asp?id=15734

43   Rose, DP; Connolly, JM. "Effects of dietary omega-3 fatty acids on human breast cancer growth and metastases in nude mice," Journal of the National Cancer Institute, 1993 Nov 3; 85(21):1743-7, found in http://www.ncbi.nlm.nih.gov/pubmed/8411258

44   Simopoulos, Artemis P., MD. "Omega-3 fatty acids in wold plants, nuts and seeds," Asia Pacific Journal of Clinical Nutrition (2002) 11(56): S163-S173.

fatty acids, can do considerable mischief. But they are not supposed to be left alone. The human evolutionary diet, and the human diet until rather recently in history, did guarantee an equal or close proportion of omega 6 fatty acids to omega 3 fatty acids. It has only been the last fifty years, or so, that government policy and crude economic logic, devoid of considerations of the health of the consumers, brought about a food production system in the United States, which also affects other countries to which we export beef or chickens, and Canada, that severely tilts the proportion in favor of omega 6.

In explaining the essential fatty acids, we considered each acid separately. Of course, as I have stated above, that the constructive, positive results of the essential fatty acids in our body is the result of omega 6 fatty acids and omega 3 fatty acids working together. Historically that has been the case. But, in very recent years, with the U.S. government subsidizing the corn growers at the level of $2.8 billion each year, making corn cheap, and subsequently the feed grain of feedlot cattle, factory farm chickens and factory farm pigs. The consequence is that bacon and eggs or corn flakes for breakfast, a chicken salad or turkey sandwich for lunch, and a hamburger or beef steak for dinner results in the diners of such fare eating corn for every meal. And add to the over generous, unwarranted subsidy for corn, the fact that the U.S. Government maintains a high tariff against the import of sugar, and corn has also been developed as the dominant sweetener in the United States, guaranteeing an even wider use of corn as food. The distribution of corn will be described in detail in Chapter 6, below.

Now corn of itself is not an unhealthy food. Humans, in the Western Hemisphere, have been eating corn (maize) for about 12,000 years, and they were healthy people. Of course they did not subsist on corn alone. They had beans, squash, meat, fish, tomatoes, and potatoes, among other items. And, although corn has a severely skewed distribution of omega 6 fatty acids in proportion to omega 3 fatty acids, it doesn't have the most severely skewed distribution. Thus, the chart immediately below indicates corn in comparison with other oils, some of which have a higher proportion of omega 6 fatty acids.

Table 1
Total Fat Content and Proportional Percentages of Other Fats in Various Foods

Food Name	Fat Content (%)	Fatty Acid Percentage of Total Oils		
		α-Linolenic Acid (Omega 3)	Linoleic Acid (Omega 6)	All Other Fatty Acids
Almond	54.2	--	17	83
Avocado	12	--	10	90
Brazil nut	66.9	--	24	76
Cashew	41.7	--	6	94
Corn	4	--	59	41
Evening Primrose	17	--	81	19
Filbert	62.4	--	16	84
Flax	35	58	14	28
Grape	20	--	71	29
Hemp seed	35	20	60	20
Safflower	59.5	--	75	25
Sesame	49.1	--	45	55
Soybean	17.7	7	50	43
Sunflower	47.3	--	65	35
Walnut	60	5	51	44

NOTE: Taken from Udo Erasmus. Fats that Heal; Fats that Kill, Table D7, p. 237

As you see in the table, although corn has 59% of total oil in linoleic acid (omega 6) and zero percentage in α-linolenic acid, evening primrose has 81% against zero; grapes, 71% – 0%; safflower, 75% – 0%; and sunflower, 65% – 0%. Hemp seed, soybean, and walnut also have higher percentages of linoleic acid, but the also have some α-linolenic acid to counterbalance it. Thus, corn is not the overall highest net percentage of linoleic acid among foods. However, in terms of consumption, how much evening primrose, grapes, safflower, and sunflower seeds are consumed in comparison with corn? And there's the problem. Because of the mindlessness of Congress and the utter lack of social and heath consciousness among the farmers, managers, and scientists of our food industry, Americans are fed a huge disproportion of corn, which is to say: linoleic acid.

We have seen above the consequences in poor health which derive from the operation of insufficiently counterbalanced arachidonic acid, which is a direct derivative of linoleic acid. The conditions listed were depression, hypertension, ischemic heart disease, cancer, rheumatoid arthritis, and immune disorder. A number of these conditions have been successfully treated with the application of systematic doses of omega 3 fatty acids.[45] This leads us to a brief discussion of the origins of human disease.

There are three things which can cause disease in humans. First, a toxin may enter the body. Toxins disrupt the absorption, transport, and metabolism of other important elements necessary for proper assimilation and digestion of nutrients.[46] If the toxin is a heavy metal, such as lead or mercury, it has the potential to be transported to the brain, where it will disrupt electrical circuits. This could lead to blindness, disruption of cognition, or other neuronic malfunction. A Toxin may also be of biological origin. One of the, if not the, most deadly such poisons is cyanide, which is produced by certain bacteria, fungi, and algae and are found in a number of plants. Once it is ingested, it attaches to the iron in the red blood cells so that oxygen cannot be carried. The cytochrome oxidase, cellular respiration, is inactivated in each cell; the cell cannot process oxygen, and dies. The death of the person, after suffering from the inability to respire, is quick. And an organism can act directly to deliver toxins in the body, such as in the case of acid tolerant Escherichia coli 0157:H7. Once ingested, this bacterium issues disruptive molecules each time it reproduces. If a minimum of 70 or 80 such bacteria are ingested, the disruption is fatal.

Toxins may come from unsuspecting sources, leading slowly to disease, which may subsequently lead to death. Hydrogenated foods, such as

---

45   Covington, Maggie B., M.D. "Omega-3 Fatty Acids," American Family Physician, July 1, 2004 found in http://www.aafp.org/afp/20040701/133.html also Rose, DP. "Effects of dietary omega-3 fatty acids on human breast cancer growth and metastases in nude mice," Journal of the National Cancer Institute, 1993 Nov 3; 85(21):1743-7, in http://www.nebi.nlm.nih.gov/pubmed/8411258 and "Omega-3 fatty acids," University of Maryland Medical Center, in http://www.umm.edu/altmed/articles/omega-3-000316.htm and Mori, Trevor A. "Omega 3 Fatty Acids and Hypertension in Humans," Clinical and Experimental Pharmacology and Physiology, Volume 33, Number 9, September 2006 , pp. 842-846(5)

46   "Sources of Heavy Metals and Chemical Toxins," http://www.hairanalysisprogram.com/articles/heavy-metals-chemical-toxin.php

margarine, contain many trans-fats, which accumulate around the heart. Continued consumption of hydrogenated fats can lead, after years, to ischemic heart disease.

The second thing which may cause disease is the attack upon the body by a pathogen. Thus, Lyme disease is caused in North America by the bacterium Borrelia burgdorferi and is transmitted to humans by the bite of infected blacklegged ticks.[47] This infection results in headaches, fatigue, and skin rashes. If untreated, it can migrate to the nerves. Another pathogen, mycobacterium tuberculosis, causes the disease tuberculosis. Tuberculosis most commonly attacks the lungs (as pulmonary TB) but can also affect the central nervous system, the lymphatic system, the circulatory system, the genitourinary system, bones, joints and even the skin.[48] Salmonella is another pathogen which attacks people. Up until several decades, it was a contractable only from turtles and other reptiles, inhabitants of wetlands.[49] Recently, it has become endemic among chickens in chicken factory farms. It passed along in factory farm eggs. And, with the commercial farm use of factory farm chicken manure fertilizer, it is also passed to consumers in commercially raised tomatoes and lettuce, foods which are usually uncooked. Salmonella causes an infection in the small intestines. It is very difficult to treat because it operates among the colony of commensal bacteria in the person's intestines. There are many other disease causing pathogens.

The third disease causing agent is a deficiency among the essential factors of physical health. These number about 50:[50]

- 2 essential fatty acids (EFAs);
- 8 essential amino acids (10 for children, 11 for premature infants);
- 13 vitamins
- 20 or 21 minerals (depending on whether tin is included);
- a source of energy (carbohydrates are the cleanest source);
- water;

---

47 "Learn about Lyme disease," Center for Disease Control (CDC), in http://www.cdc.gov/ncidod/dvbid/lyme/index.htm

48 http://en.wikipedia.org/wiki/Tuberculosis

49 http://en.wikipedia.org/wiki/Salmonella

50 Slightly adapted from Udo Erasmus. Fats that Heal; Fats that Kill, 1993 (2nd ed.), pp. 73-74.

- oxygen; and
- light.

One deficiency disease is scurvy, which used to affect seamen on long sea voyages in the eighteenth and early nineteenth centuries. We now know that it is caused by a deficiency of Vitamin C. A deficiency of Vitamin B_3 causes pellagra, and beriberi is the result of a deficiency of Vitamin B_1. A deficiency in Vitamin D can cause hypertension and reduced immunity function. Iron deficiency can lead to fatigue and other conditions. We can discuss other types of deficiency conditions, but in this extended essay we will focus on diseases derivative of deficiencies in the essential fatty acids (EFAs).

There are two EFAs which are made by plants, but which we cannot make, and, therefore, must be attained by consuming plants or plant eating animals. These are alpha-linolenic acid (omega 3 fatty acid) and linoleic acid (omega 6 fatty acid). In Table 1 above you can see that flax, hemp seed, soybean, and walnuts all have alpha-linolenic acid. Other seed oils with the omega 3 fatty acid are chia, pumpkin, wheat germ, and rape seed (canola). Alpha-linolenic acid is more easily gotten from the consumption of green, leafy vegetables and whole grains. Because linoleic acid (omega 6 fatty acid) is more persistent, it is present in all of the seed oils, and in many vegetables and fruits also. Human health requires that there be a balance between these to EFAs in the human diet. That balance should consist of an omega 6 to omega 3 fatty acid ratio range of from 1:2 to 4:1. Outside of that range, in a persisting diet, human health is threatened.

Because of the widespread use of corn as the dominant grain in the food for beef cattle, swine, and chickens, both layers and broilers, as well as the use of corn in breakfast cereals, the omega 6 to omega 3 fatty acid ratio of many American ranges from 10:1 to 40:1. This explains why the United States is the across the board world leader in the proportion of people suffering from depression, rheumatoid arthritis, hypertension, ischemic heart disease mortality, breast cancer, and others. A dubious distinction, it is the cost of the consumption of so much corn.

Before continuing the discussion of the health consequences of the disproportionate amount of omega 6 fatty acids in the American diet, it should be stated that the degeneration into atherosclerosis and ischemic heart disease is a result of the disproportionate arachidonic acid in the body, as well as other deficiencies, including all or some of vitamins C, A, E, B_6, B_3, B_2, and folic acid, as well as deficiencies in iodine, manganese, copper, chromium, and selenium. Nationwide dietetic surveys have found that 60% of the people in North America are deficient in one or more essential nutrients,[51] probably among those listed in the previous sentence. Severe deficiency diseases are usually the result of more than one deficiency; however, the focus of this essay is on the deficiency of omega 3 fatty acids, and the disproportionate consumption of omega 6 fatty acids produced by the disproportionate consumption of corn. It should also be noted that corn, unlike any other grain, is deficient in Niacin,[52] Vitamin B_3; so, an over reliance on corn in one's diet could also result in a deficiency in this vitamin. The deficiency represented by the disproportionate consumption of omega 6 fatty acids, even if it does not act alone in the development of a severe disease, is always a major player.

The omega 6 fatty acid, arachidonic acid, has been found to support dermal integrity, renal function, and parturition in human development.[53] However, when there is a large ratio of omega 6 fatty acids to omega 3 fatty acids the physiological state in the tissues is shifted toward the pathogenesis of many diseases: prothrombotic, proinflammatory, and proconstrictive.[54] So, chronic excessive production of the omega 6 long chain fatty acid, arachidonic acid, not countered with omega 3 fatty acids, is associated with arthritis, heart attacks, thrombotic stroke, arrhythmia, osteoporosis, inflammation, mood disorders, and cancer.[55]

As indicated above, one of three long chained polyunsaturated acid derivatives of linoleic acid is arachidonic acid. In small doses, counterbalanced with an almost equal number of omega 3 acids, arachidonic acid is very beneficial to human development and physiological maintenance. In large does, compared to omega 3 acids, arachidonic acid is disruptive and harmful. In proper small doses it maintains dermal integrity; in large,

---

51   Erasmus, Udo. Fats that Heal; Fats that Kill, p. 180

52   http://en.wikipedia.org/wiki/Niacin

53   http://en.wikipedia.org/wiki/Omega-3_fatty_acid

54   Simopoulos, Artemis P. (September 2003) "Importance of the ratio of omega-6/omega-3 essential fatty acids evolutionary aspects," World Review of Nutrition and Dietetics, p. 92.

55   Calder, Philip C. (June 2006). "n-3 polyunsaturated fatty acids, inflammation, and inflammatory diseases," American Journal of Clinical Nutrition 83, pp. 1505s-1519s; http://cancerres.aacrjournals.org/cgi/content/text/48/23/6642; and http://www.news-medical.net/print_article.asp?id=15734

uncounterbalanced doses, it causes tumors.[56] Arachidonic acid, along with the other omega 6 acids, contributes to autoimmune diseases, including arthritis, Crohn's disease, ulcerative colitis, and lupus erythematosis.[57] Arachidonic acid travels to, and is a normal complement of the chemistry of, the brain. But in large doses it affects moods, attention spans, and the bipolar disorder.[58] Attention deficit disorder in children is probably attributable to large quantities of arachidonic acid in their brain. And there has been a study linking omega 6 derivative acids to depression.[59]

A chronic and potentially disabling autoimmune disorder is rheumatoid arthritis, the prevalence rate of which in the United States is 1%, "...with women affected three to five times as often as men."[60] Table 2, immediately below, shows the average prevalence rate, for both men and women, for 16 European countries. The date of the data and the age group from which the data were drawn are provided.

Table 2
Prevalence of Rheumatoid Arthritis from Individual Studies Across Europe

Country (Ordered North to South)	Year(s) Data were gathered	Age Group	Prevalence Percentage
Iceland	1974-83	39-67	0.24
Finland	1989	≥16	0.8
Norway	1994	20-79	0.43
Sweden	1965-67	31-74	0.27
Russia	1999	≥20	1.42
Denmark	?	≥15	0.6

56   "Fatty acids such as those found in corn oil turn on genes that stimulate tumor growth," NEWS-MEDICAL.NET, found in http://www.news-medical.net/print_article.asp?id=15734

57   Simopoulos, AP. "Omega-3 acids in inflammation and autoimmune diseases," Journal of the American College of Nutrition, 2002 Dec 21(6), pp. 495-505

58   Lee, H. J.; Rao, J.S.; Rapoport, S.I.; Bazinet, R. P. (November 2007) "Antimanic therapies target brain arachidonic acid signaling, Lessons learned about the regulation of grain fatty acid metabolism," Prostaglandins, Leukotrienes and Essential Fatty Acids, 77(5): 239-246. Elsevier

59   http://en.wikipedia.org/wiki/Fatty_acid

60   http://en.wikipedia.org/wiki/Rheumatodid_arthritis

Table 2
Prevalence of Rheumatoid Arthritis from Individual Studies Across Europe

Country (Ordered North to South)	Year(s) Data were gathered	Age Group	Prevalence Percentage
UK	2000	≥16	0.8
Czech Republic	1965	≥15	0.4
Germany	1990	≥20	0.83
France	1996	≥18	0.59
Slovakia	1970's	≥35	1.3
Italy	1991-92	≥16	0.7
Yugoslavia	1990-91	≥20	0.19
Bulgaria	1965	≥15	0.75
Spain	2000	≥20	0.5
Greece	1967-95	≥16	0.35

SOURCE: "Indicators for Monitoring Musculoskeletal Conditions Project," European Commission, Health & Consumer Protection Directorate, Directorate C - Public Health and Risk Assessment, Table 7.

As can be seen, all of the prevalence rates, with the exception of the one for Russia and the one for Slovakia, are below the United States rate of 1.0. But comparing the United States with those countries with comparable lifestyles, the Scandinavian countries and the states of western Europe, the Unites States' prevalence rate is higher than all of those. Why should it be so high? Is it a deficient medical service? No, we are among the best trained and equipped in the world. Is it genetic? But the majority of our populations shares close genes with Europeans. Again, the culprit seems to be the great disproportion of arachidonic acid in our population because of the near ubiquity of corn.

Excess arachidonic acid, derivative from the consumption of an excessive proportion of omega 6 fatty acids, as compared to omega 3 fatty acids, will also cause the clumping of blood platelets, and contribute to the narrowing of arteries and high blood pressure. About 25% of all Americans suffer from high blood pressure.[61] About one-third of the people suffering from high blood pressure, which has no symptoms, are unaware of their

---

61   From the National Heart, Lung, and Blood Institute website at http://www.nhlbi.nih.gov/hbp/intro.htm

condition.[62] Persistent high blood pressure can lead to renal failure, and, more frequently, to heart attack (myocardial infarction). The World Health Organization (WHO) estimated that, in 2002, 12.6% of deaths worldwide were from ischemic heart disease, the common presentation of myocardial infarction, commonly referred to as coronary heart attack.[63] In the United States coronary heart attack is the leading cause of death, accounting for 20% of U.S. premature deaths.

Now we may ask why one-fourth of all Americans suffer from high blood pressure. There are a number of possible contributors, including tension, persistent overexertion, salt intolerance. But these could not account for fully one-fourth of all Americans. But diet, particularly the excessive consumption of omega 6 fatty acids could, and given the typical American diet, it probably is the leading cause of high blood pressure.

How can we account for the fact that Americans suffer death by heart attack so much more frequently than do people worldwide? Fully one-fifth, 20%, of all Americans suffer death by heart attach annually, whereas the same cause accounts for 12.6% of deaths worldwide. Again, what is the peculiarity of the American experience? It is the consumption of a great deal of corn. It is done through the consumption of feedlot beef, swine, and factory farm chicken, factory farm chicken eggs, as well as many other food items, which will be discussed below. But the consumption of corn, as in corn fed beef, leading to the production of excessive arachidonic acid is probably the cause of as many as half of the heart attacks suffered by Americans.

The disproportionate consumption of omega 6 fatty acid has also been linked to breast cancer.[64] The incidence evidence again points to the peculiar corn diet of the United States. The table below, in twelve world regions, indicates the annual age-standardized incidence rates of breast cancer per 100,000 women.

---

62   http://www.americanheart.org/presenter.jhtml?identifier=2114

63   http://en.wikipedia.org/wiki/Heart_attacks

64   Rose DP and Connolly JM. "Effects of dietary omega-3 fatty acids on human breast cancer growth and metastases in nude mice," National Cancer Institute 1993 Nov 3;85(21):1743-7 retrieved in http://www.ncbi.nlm.nhih.gov/pubmed/8411258

Table 3

**Annual Incidence of Breast Cancer per 100,000 Women
Age-Standardized Rates**

Region	Average Rate
Eastern Asia	18
South Central Asia	22
Sub-Saharan Africa	22
South-Eastern Asia	26
North Africa and Western Asia	28
South and Central America	42
Eastern Europe	49
Southern Europe	56
Northern Europe	73
Oceania	74
Western Europe	78
North America	90
NOTE: Data derived from http://wikipedia.org/wiki/Breast_cancer	

Again, the region in which the United States is, and is the major population, has the highest average annual incidence of all the twelve regions. What makes the region of the United States peculiar? It is not wealth; northern and western Europe are also wealthy. Is it our mix of different ethnicities? But all of our ethnicities, except for native Americans, come from some other region of the world, and all of the other regions of the world have lower annual average incidence. No, the peculiarity of the United States is its corn diet, corn-fed beef, pork, and chicken, as well as the other food item which we will discuss below. Excessive proportion of omega 6 fatty acids, and arachidonic acid in particular, are probably responsible for at least a quarter, and probably much more, of the annual cases of breast cancer in the United States.

The first two definitions of "poison" by the American Heritage Dictionary are "1. A substance that causes injury, illness, or death, esp. by chemical means. 2. Something that is destructive or fatal."[65] Certainly, corn fed beef, swine, and chickens are destructive and all too often fatal. And

---

65   The American Heritage Dictionary, Second College Edition.

it can also be argued that the artificial feeding of these feed stock animals are the chemical means to cause injury, illness, or death for American consumers. By either definition, it can be said that the United States, since the middle of the last century, has devised a food system which is poisoning Americans.

We will now discuss, in some detail, how this malicious food is grown and developed.

3 - The Production of Beef

CATTLE FEEDLOTS

DATA FROM THE U.S. Department of Agriculture indicate that, at the beginning of April 2003 cattle and calves for slaughter on feedlots with a capacity of 1,000 or more head totaled 10.7 million. Of the total feedlot inventory, steer and steer calves accounted for 63 percent, or 6.72 million. Heifers and heifer calves totaled 3.92 million. Three states dominated cattle feedlot production: Texas had 2.7 million cattle on feedlots; Kansas, 2.3 million; and Nebraska, 2.2 million. These three states accounted for two-thirds of all beef cattle feedlot production, and large feedlot production accounted for one-third (10.7 million) of the 33 million beef cattle in the United States in April of 2003.[66]

THE CORN DIET

BEFORE AND DURING THE Second World War (1938-45, 1941-45 for the U.S.A.) all cattle were raised on pasture land. Milk cows and their calves were raised on pastures, as many still are. Steers and heifers, raised for beef, were also raised on pastures. It took two to three years for a steer or a heifer to attain the weight which made it profitable to slaughter. And there was no E-coli 0157:H7 poisoning problem. All cattle have E-coli bacteria in their digestive system. But, as has been explained above, when cattle are grass fed, as their bodies have been evolved to do, their digestive tract, as well as the E-coli within it, is PH neutral, and cannot harm a person eating such

66   http://www.answers.com/topic/beef-cattle-feedlots?cat=biz-fin

a grass fed steer. Bacteria, including E-coli, are very tiny, much smaller than a human cell. When slaughtering and butchering a steer, it is very difficult to prevent E-coli, and other bacteria, from getting on the beef. But if it is a grass fed steer or heifer, there is no harm, there are absolutely no consequences, from ingesting such E-coli along the beef. Even today, if you eat beef from a steer or heifer which has been pasture raised, there is no danger from ingesting its E-coli. E-coli 0157:H7, which is an acid tolerant bacterium, and which is poisonous for humans to consume, does not develop in a grass fed steer or heifer.[67]

After the Second World War the U.S. feedlot method of raising steers and heifers for slaughter began. It was a result of a coincidence of several developments. The stock pile of left over nitrate material for explosives making was now available for fertilizer. This promoted the growth and yields of corn on the Great Plains. It also required the increased pumping of water from the Ogallala Aquifer. A second development was antibiotics. This would allow the close quartering of cattle without the fear of them getting ill. A third development was the production of vitamins, particularly Vitamin D, which would allow the housing of cattle for extended periods without the fear of illness from vitamin deficiency. But the cost for these, and for hormonal additives developed later, was justified by the reduction of the fattening time to get the steers and heifers ready for slaughter, from two to three years on pasture, to 14 months in a feedlot.

Factory farms, including feedlots, also known as Concentrated Animal Feeding Operations (CAFOs), also developed in Europe. The basic feed of the European steer raisers was hay and straw. In the United States, with its abundantly subsidized corn,[68] and its abundantly free water from the Ogallala Aquifer, the basic feed of feedlot cattle is corn.

But the feeding of cattle with corn is a major problem. Cattle, members of the family Bovidae, were evolved, and have the digestive system, to eat only grass. Certainly, when eating grass, cattle sometimes ingest grass seeds. With the blades of grass the primary food, these small quantities of grass seed pass right through. Feeding only corn and some other grains to cattle, however, presents a problem. Corn has a large proportion of starch, which needs to be broken down, in the short time it has in the animal's digestive system, acidicly. Humans can eat corn safely; our acidic digestive

---

67 http://en.wikipedia.org/wiki/Cattle_feeding

68 http://en.wiki pedia.org/wiki/Agricultural_subsidy

system breaks it down and converts it to sugar and fat. If a steer or heifer is to survive on a diet of corn, and a number of them do not, then it has to develop an acidic process to break it down. Escherichia coli is a bacterium in all mammals which processes food. The normal cattle E-coli, which normally engages a fermentation process to digest grass, cannot function, cannot survive, in an acidic environment. Thus the E-coli of cattle who do survive on corn have to revert to an atavistic form[69] to become the acid resistant E-coli 0157:H7. If, then, in eating the muscle fiber of a corn fed steer, some E-coli 0157:H7 is ingested by a human, the bacterium would survive the human acid stomach. With no role in a human digestive system, it essentially disrupts the system by releasing molecules when it reproduces, which molecules are toxic to humans, and the consequence is that the human becomes ill. If a large enough number of such E-coli 0157:H7 are ingested, the disruption and toxicity will be of such magnitude that the human consumer dies.

Thus, corn fed beef is dangerous, and potentially lethal, to consume. Its main hazard, as explained just above, is the presence of E-coli 0157:H7 bacteria in beef. Although food borne bacteria can be killed simply by thoroughly heating the meat to at least 160°F (71.1°C), this is evidently not always done.

> The bacteria, E. Coli 0157:H7, killed four people who ate hamburgers at fast-food restaurants in four Western states last year [1993], sickened more than 700 and sent 178 to hospitals.[70]

So, in the initial ten years, or so, of distributing corn-fed beef, an estimated over 50 people died from E-coli 0157:H7 poisoning. People during this time, as well as before and after, who ate only grass fed beef did not, could not, get E-coli 0157:H7 poisoning. None of them died from eating their grass fed beef.

---

69   I am hypothesizing that there are still provisions in the E-coli DNA for it to function acidicly. These would relate to a time, millions of years ago, when its host was either carnivorous or a consumer of complex carbohydrates. A fetal dolphin has vestigial legs. Evidently, the dolphin DNA retains instructions on the making of legs. This refers to a time millions of years ago. Chickens still have instructions in their DNA to make teeth. Again, this refers to a time millions of years ago. These two examples, plus the fact that the acid tolerant E-coli 0157:H7 is common in all surviving grain fed cattle, support my hypothesis of reversion.

70   The New York Times, July 14, 1994, p. 1.

Something had to be done to reduce this human engineered danger. In July 1994, a panel of Federal, industry, and health officials strongly recommended the irradiation of at least some beef, particularly ground beef.[71] By 1994, irradiation was approved for the use for pork to control Trichina. The FDA had also approved the irradiation of poultry.[72] Now, before the year 2000, irradiation meant dosing the food with gamma rays derivative of a radioactive substance, usually Cobalt-80, or Cobalt-60. When irradiating food with radioactive Cobalt-80, or Cobalt-60, molecules called 'radiotoxines' are formed and left in the food. Among these radiotoxines are formaldehyde and benzene, both of which are carcinogenic. The FDA refers to these radiotoxines as 'radiolytic by-products.'[73] By mid 2000 a method of electronic irradiation was approved. This method used no radioactive materials. Instead, it bombards the food with a very high energy beam of electrons by the use of x-rays. This causes the destruction of the DNA (Deoxyribonucleic Acid) of virtually all of the cells in the food. The destruction of the residual DNA of the dead steer muscle produces no adverse consequences, other than reducing the number of usable nutrients in the beef. But the method also destroys the DNA of the E-coli 0157:H7, and that makes the meat safe from E-coli 0157:H7 poisoning, even if not heated sufficiently. Because of the damage to vitamins, it is also less nutritious to eat.

So, irradiated beef is safe, that is, from E-coli 0157:H7. But corn fed beef is unhealthy, to the point that it is unsafe, for the severe imbalance it creates for omega fatty acids. Fifteen years later, to possibly avoid the cost or inconvenience of electronic processing, producers of ground beef, which included the swept up fat trimmings, added ammonia to kill the E-coli 0157:H7. Some of that ammonia remained in the beef patties.

During human evolution the foods that were eaten maintained a close ration of omega 6 and omega 3 fatty acids. The antelope, and later, cows humans ate subsisted on grass. The meat of grass fed cows, or antelope, has an omega 6 to omega 3 fatty acid ratio of between 1:1 to 2:1.[74] The whole grain seeds, and fruits and nuts humans would have eaten are also rich in omega 3 fatty acids. And it may be said that until the midpoint

71 *Idem.*

72 http://www.maine.gov/education/sfs/irrbeef.html

73 http://www.liferesearchuniversal.com/radiation.html

74 2005 British Society for Immunology,Clinical and Experimental Immunology,142: p. 217

of the twentieth century, the chickens, pork, and beef the people of the United States ate had a close ratio of omega 6 to omega 3 fatty acids, consistent with human evolutionary experience. Since that time, a very large proportion of the typical American diet contains a large proportion of corn, and the animals raised for meat are all fed large quantities of corn. And corn, as has been demonstrated above, is a peculiar grain in that it contains practically no omega 3 fatty acids, and a large proportion of omega 6 fatty acids. The near ubiquity of corn in the American food supply will be discussed below in Chapter 6, but for now it should be mentioned that a very high proportion of Americans consume omega 6 to omega 3 fatty acid ratios in the range of 30:1 to 40:1. Ratios of over 4:1 may be considered excessive.

We are not through with cattle and the production of beef in CAFOs. We have only, thus far, discussed the effects of the use of corn as the main ingredient of cattle feed; there are other deleterious things that are added to that feed, which we will discuss immediately below. But you can already see that corn fed beef is not safe to eat.

THE USE OF ANTIBIOTICS

IN 2001, THE UNION of Concerned Scientists estimated that greater than 70% of the antibiotics used in the United States are given to food animals, chickens, pigs, and cattle, in the absence of disease.[75] Well, if you are going to crowd 80 to 150 cattle in extremely close quarters, where they have to stand and rest in their own collective feces, you have created a disease generation system. The concern is the contraction of campylobacter infection and coccidiosis. These diseases are quite rare in pasture raised cattle. They are, however, a concern in feedlots.[76] These diseases are transmitted by the ingestion of infected feces, a circumstance that, you may assume, occurs frequently in feedlots. So, in 1951 the FDA approved the use of antibiotics in animal feed without a veterinary medical prescription.

Such indiscriminate use of antibiotics are bound to have effects, including, perhaps, those not anticipated by the authorities. Antibiotics put stress on pathogenic bacteria. The intended effect is for the stress to be lethal. To be sure, that is the effect on most of the pathogenic bacteria. Some strains of bacteria may be all killed out, but other strains may have

---

75   Reported in http://en.wikipedia.org/wiki/Antibiotic_resistance

76   http://en.wikipedia.org/wiki/Cattle_feeding

a few survivors. That's the way evolution works. Those who can survive in a new, hostile environment are the ones who produce progeny. While campylobacter, which form in cattle is species specific, may have been largely controlled, if not momentarily eliminated in cattle, it is unlikely it is eliminated.

Feedlot owners are also secure in their use of antibiotics because the antibiotics they use are approved by the Food and Drug Administration (FDA). But the FDA is not known to have ever refused a request from a pharmaceutical company for use of one of its antibiotics in animal feed. They seem to be brought to deny the use of an antibiotic only after antibiotic resistance has occurred. And, although the FDA has the authority to approve and regulate the use of nontherapeutic levels of antibiotics in animal feed, there is no U.S. data collection system regarding the specific types and amounts of antibiotics that are used for this purpose.[77]

Not only is there no U.S. data collection on the use of antibiotics on factory farms, the state governments, which are primarily responsible for their residents health under the U.S. Constitution, also collect no data with respect to antibodies, or any drug use. It is not as though the drugs used on factory farms are distinct from those used by humans.

Many of these antibiotics are the same compounds that are administered to humans in clinical setting, and include tetracyclines, macrolides, strepotgramins, and fluoroquinolones.[78]

So, pathogenic bacteria are becoming resistant to antibiotics. Not only to veterinary specific medications, but to the very antibiotics used for human patients in hospitals. "Since 1976 several persuasive scientific studies have illustrated how animals fed low-dose antibiotics not only propagate resistant bacteria, but spread these resistant strains to farmers, their families, community residents, and ultimately, hospitalized patients."[79] This may be characterized as unhealthy, but it is also socially dangerous. It could also be individually dangerous to an American eating a fairly typical American

77 Sapkota, Amy R., Lefferts, Lisa Y., Mckenzie, Shawn, and Walker, Polly. "What Do We Feed to Food-Production Animals? A Review of Animal Feed Ingredients and Their Potential Impacts on Human Health," Environmental Health Perspectives, Vol. 115, No. 5 (May 2007), p. 665.

78 Idem.

79 Bonnie M. Marshall and Stuart B. Levy, "Antibiotics in the Animals We Eat," The Scientist, April 1, 2012.

diet, with bacon and eggs for breakfast, from a corn fed swine and from corn fed chickens, and a dinner of beef steak, rare, from a corn fed steer. And, of course, a salad to go with the dinner. A disease, such as campylobacter jejuni, which has become fluoroquinolone-resistant,[80] could have been contracted from the pork or the chickens, and the lettuce fertilized with beef manure, could land that American in a hospital, with few or no medications available to treat the condition. A very unhealthy condition, all courtesy of the American factory farm system of meat production.

THE USE OF HORMONES

INFORMATION ABOUT HORMONE ADMINISTRATION to food production cattle at U.S. CAFOs is not readily available. The cattle feed producers or the CAFOs are not forthcoming about the inclusion of hormones in cattle feed, or the administration of hormones by some other method. But, by indirect methods, some estimates of types, more than quantities, of hormones used have been made. At the start of 1989, the European banned beef to which any of a list of hormones had been given.[81] This began a ban on American beef imports, which in 1989 was valued at $130 million. The hormones listed were:[82]

- estradiol
- progesterone
- testosterone
- melengesterol acetate
- trenbolone acetate, and
- zeranol

The Europeans asserted that they opposed the use of hormones because it is part of a system of feed-lot abuse, that the hormones are used to get unnatural, quick growth. The Europeans claim to want a more natural setting. Of course it was left unsaid that the European production of beef also involved feed-lots. But, in fairness, it should be mentioned that the ban applied to Europe as well as other countries, including the United States.

---

80   *Ibid.*, p. 667

81   Freudenheim, Milt. "Beef Dispute: Stakes High in Trade War," The New York Times, January 1, 1989, p. 1.

82   http:/en.wikipedia.org/wiki/Beef_hormone_controversy

The New York Times article cited above also reports an interview with Tommy R. Beal, who, in 1989, was Market Research Director at Cattle-Fax, a service affiliated with the National Cattlemen's Association. Mr. Beal was reported to have said that without the hormones, the cost of adding 400 pounds to a steer or heifer before slaughter would raise the costs by $20. To put that figure in the context of the whole cattle industry, he said that the hormone implants save the industry at least $650 million a year.

A hormone implant, which costs the feed lot operator one dollar each, is implanted 120 days before slaughter. Not only does it save $20 in fattening costs, but it also cuts the feeding period by 18 days. This increases the number of cattle the feed lot can handle each year. The hormones also make for 50 more pounds in lean meat. Between 70 and 90 per cent of all feed lot cattle receive hormone implants.

Hormone implants also make feed lot cattle easier to handle. "The hormones have a calming effect, basically desexing the animals so that more of them can raised in confined areas," said Dr. Lester M. Crawford, head of the Agricultural Department's Food Safety and Inspection Service.[83]

But we are interested in the health implications of this practice rather than its financial aspects. In this regard, estradiol, progesterone, melengesterol acetate, and zeranol are all female sex hormones. Estradiol is estrogen in a mammal's system. Estrogen is also a hormone in a male body, where it promotes bone growth and bone strength. But the hormone plays a much larger role in a female body. Progesterone is a steroid hormone which regulates the menstrual cycle in human females, and plays a role in gestation. Melengesterol acetate is used to synchronize estrus in cattle. It also is related to the processing and building of fat. And zeranol is a synthetic non-steroidal estrogenic growth promoter.[84] These hormones do not get into the muscle fiber, the meat, but they do pass in the feces of the animals. This puts a disproportionate amount of female hormones in the environment.

On December 19, 2003 Edward Orlando, Assistant Professor of biology at St. Mary's College of Maryland, reported the findings of his group, which involved a study of minnows in three streams that flow into Nebraska's Elkhorn River. They found "significant alterations in

83 Freudenheim, Milt. "Beef Dispute: Stakes High In Trade War," The New York Times, January 1, 1989, p. 1.

84 "Drugs and Health Products: Proposal for Zeranol," found in http://www.hc-cs. gc.ca/dhp-mps/vet/mrl-lmr_zeranol-eng.php

the reproductive biology" of fish immediately downstream from a large Nebraska cattle feedlot.[85]

The scientists further reported that they do not know whether the damage was caused by natural hormones in cattle or by synthetic one administered to the animals. Their report states that the findings clearly demonstrate that effluent from feedlots is hormonally active, whether it is natural or synthetic. About 30 million head of cattle are raised in U.S. feedlots each year, and nearly all are implanted with growth-promoting synthetic hormones.[86]

Thus, the indiscriminate use of hormones has already altered the environment in streams, at least those relatively close to feedlots. The minnow study was in 2003. Might the hormone pollution have continued downstream since then? Adversely affecting the environment this way has the potential of adversely affecting many species, including humans.

OTHER ITEMS

THE FEED GIVEN FEEDLOT cattle contains more than only grains and antibiotics. Voicing the absolutely nonsensical mantra, "protein is protein," and "fat is fat," feed preparers added rendered meat, chicken litter, beef tallow, dried cow milk, and dried cow blood to cattle feed. Mindful of the need for fibre in the diet, preparers also add sand, wood, and even plastics.

In the 1980s " Mad Cow Disease" (Bovine Spongiform Encephalopathy, BSE) came on the international scene, first being detected in Britain. The cause was agreed to be the feeding of meat to cattle. In Britain it was the feeding of rendered goats or sheep with scrapie, a spongiform encephalopathy. Careful analysis then identified the pathogenic agent as a prion. This is a misshapen protein which is passed from a diseased animal to another by ingestion. In 1986 the first cases of BSE were described in Britain; in 1988 the feeding of rendered meat to cattle was banned.[87] In

85   "SMCM professor discovers cattle hormones that leak into streams and alter fish reproduction," 19.12.2003, found in http://www.innovations-report.com/html/environment_sciences/Report-24374.html

86   *Idem.*

87   Norris, Sonya. "Bovine Spongiform Encephalopathy and its Relationship with Jakob-Creutzfeldt Desease," [Canadian] Library of Parliament, Parliamentary Research and Information Service, 20 January 2004, found in http://www.parl.gc.ca/information/library/PRBpubs/prb0327-e.htm

the first week of January 2000 the European Union banned the inclusion of meat in the feeding cattle throughout Europe.[88]

What has been the response of the United States? From the same minds which generated "protein is protein" and "fat is fat," the decision was made to stop the feeding of only rendered beef meat to cattle; beef meat and others could still be fed to swine and chickens, and cattle could still eat the rendered meat of butcher shops, supermarkets, restaurants, fast-food chains, poultry processors, slaughterhouses, farms, ranches, feedlots, and animal shelters,[89] exclusive only of cattle meat. In 2003 one case of BSE was found in the United States. Careful analysis revealed that the affected cow had eaten contaminated food. The contamination occurred because of the carelessness of the food preparer making cattle feed in the same mixing vats used to made the feed for swine and chickens. With the reputation and sales of the CAFO beef industry in jeopardy, the preparers were strongly urged to segregate the feed preparation processes. In the following five years there has been no case of BSE among feedlot cattle.

So, now, if the reader has been eating feedlot beef, she or he will now know how that beef has been raised. These animals, which evolved as grazing animals, are feed a largely corn diet, admixed with antibiotics; sand, sawdust, and ground plastic; and the rendered meat of a variety of animals. Nothing about the raising of these animals has been healthy, and eating of the resulting beef is unhealthy, and, in the case of antibiotic resistant bacteria, dangerous.

THE COST TO HUMANS OF FEEDLOT BEEF

THE COST TO AMERICANS and to American society of feedlot beef is great. Starting with the grain fed to the cattle. It is mostly corn. And corn is peculiar in that it has a disproportionate amount of omega 6 (Linoleic acid) fatty acid. The proportion, as expressed in the proportion of omega 6 to omega 3 is about 46:1. As has been said above, omega 6 fatty acid is one of the two essential fatty acids required in the diet of humans, because we cannot make these acids ourselves. The other is omega 3 (α-Linolenic acid) fatty acid. Without linoleic acid (omega 6) a human could not survive. Linoleic acid, itself and in its derivative acids, is essential to the formation

---

88   http://www.democracynow.org/2000/12/6/europe_bans_meat_based_cattle_feed

89   http://www.epa.gov/ttn/chief/ap42/ch09/final/c9s05-3.pdf

of cell and organelle membranes, and the formation and strengthening of arterial and veined structures. A derivative acid, Arachidonic acid, contributes to this structural building and is essential for the functioning of the brain.

But, the omega 6 and derivative acids are, after all, mindless acids, and the constructive deeds of omega 6 acids are dependent on their counterbalance with α-linolenic acid (omega 3), and its derivatives. This counterbalance has to be pretty close. In our recent evolution, and even now, the eating of grass fed cattle renders an omega 6 to omega 3 ratio of about 1:1 or 2:1, and the traditional human diet, in is variations, has ranged from 4:1 to 1:2.5. Human health, mental and physical, can be maintained by a balanced diet respecting that range. But with corn-fed beef, as well as corn in so many commercial food products, the American ratio has been between 20:1 and 40:1. This is exceedingly unhealthy, and is responsible, as detailed above, for much of the disease, including neoplasms, high blood pressure, heart attacks, breast cancer, bi-polar syndrome, and AHD, and premature death. Corn-fed beef is part of this syndrome. And part of its cost to Americans is the amount of suffering and lost time because of disease and premature death.

Corn-fed cattle are also responsible for other deaths. The feeding of corn and other grains, as well as rendered meat, had forced the originally neutral E-coli intestinal bacterium of feedlot cattle to revert to its very ancient form, when its host was grain eating, to what is now labeled E-coli 0157:H7. This is its acid tolerant form which is toxic to humans. Before irradiation started in 1994, 50 people were killed by the consumption of feedlot beef laden with E-coli 0157:H7. Then, between 1994 and 2000, during which time radioactive Cobalt 80 or 60 were used to irradiate beef, carcinogenic substances were produced in the irradiated beef. Only since the advent of electronic irradiation in 2000 has there been a safe way to irradiate feedlot beef with respect to E-coli 0157:H7 and carcinogens, but electronic irradiation eliminate most, if not all, of the nutrients of the beef. Yet even control of E-coli l0157:H7 is not complete. Evidently, not all feedlot beef preparers use irradiation, for there are still occasional reports of people dying from eating insufficiently cooked feedlot hamburger.

Beyond the problem of contaminated E-coli 0157:H7 beef, there is E-coli 0157:H7 contaminated manure. As is true for all mammals, intestinal bacteria are emitted in feces. In fact, a majority of the dry mass of the feces of most mammals consists of intestinal bacteria. So, there is nothing unusual for cattle who have E-coli 0157:H7 in their systems to emit the same in their manure. But it is a mindless and irresponsible practice for this manure to be sold to, and bought, by commercial vegetable and fruit farmers. In September and October of 2006 the U.S. FDA announced a "Nation-wide Outbreak of E-coli 0157:H7" in leafy greens.[90] This slightly over speaks the event. Consumers of leafy greens from local farms, particularly organic local farms, never experienced any E-coli 0157:H7 contamination. But, for most Americans, the warning was apt. From time to time there were warnings about other vegetables. And, occasionally, people have sickened and died. All is attributable to feedlot cattle. The cost is mounting up.

There is an indeterminate cost of administering hormones to the vast majority of feedlot cattle. Most of these hormones are female hormones, and it has already been found to have altered the sex of downstream fish. As Omaha and other cities draw their drinking water from the river, the consequences of waterborne hormones may potentially have, or may already be having, an effect on people.

Finally, there is the inclusion in feedlot cattle feed of rendered meat and artificial substitutes for fiber. The potential exists, of the acquisition of Jakob-Creutzfeldt Disease among consumers of such beef, although, to date, no such cases have been identified. However, the British experience tells us that it takes ten full years for unambiguous symptoms of the disease to express themselves.

Also, among the rendered meat products are the remains of dogs and cats, as well as chickens, and swine. Add to this the inclusion of sawdust and ground plastic, and such a diet produces the feeling of disgust. "Disgust" derives from the Latin "des," not, and "gustus," taste, eat. It has evolved to also mean repugnance excited by something offensive. Indeed, feedlot beef should not be eaten for this, as well as for personal and social health reasons.

---

90   U.S. Food and Drug Administration.   "Nationwide E. Coli O157:H7 Outbreak:Questions & Answers" September and October 2006, found in http://www.cfsan.fda.gov/~dms/spinacqa.html

4 - The Production of Poultry

The Origin of the Domesticated Chicken, and Their Traditional Use

The chicken (Gallus gallus, sometimes G. Gallus domesticus) is a domesticated fowl likely descended from the wild Indian and southeast Asian Red Junglefowl (Gallus gallus) and the related Grey Junglefowl (G. Sonneratii). It was long assumed that the chicken is solely descended from the Asian Red Junglefowl, and it shares many characteristics and genes with that species. However, chickens have yellow skin, but the Red Junglefowl does not, nor does it have a gene for yellow skin. The chicken's gene for yellow skin is shared only with the Grey Junglefowl. Therefore, it is now accepted that the chicken shares inheritance from both the Grey and Red Junglefowls.[91]

The diet of the Red Jungle Fowl, and probably also for the Grey Junglefowl, consists of seeds, buds, fruit, and insects.[92] They have powerful leg and toe muscles for birds, and forage for insects by scratching the forest ground.

Traditionally, before the twentieth century, farm chicken flocks tended to be small. Chickens were generally allowed out in a fenced yard, where they scratched for bugs. A flock of hens, with, perhaps a single rooster, were kept primarily for eggs, and good laying chickens laid eggs for three seasons, resting, and not laying, in the winter. This is what was meant by " kept for eggs." Because they were kept for eggs, the eating of chicken was

91   http://en.wikipedia.org/wiki/Chicken

92   http://www.encyclopedia.com/doc/1E1-junglefo.html

a rare event. When a clutch of chicks was hatched, the excess roosters were slaughtered after six or eight weeks. Otherwise, a chicken was taken for food only after she had stopped laying eggs, which was at about six years. Occasionally, a hen would stop prematurely, in which case it was considered "sick," but still considered appropriate to eat. A legend also originated in eastern Europe that if a person found him or herself sick, eating chicken, or more specifically, chicken soup, was considered the universal remedy. Thus, the aphorism arose in Jewish east European villages that if a man were to be seen eating a chicken, one of them was presumed sick.

So, while eggs were readily available, for three seasons, in small villages and on small farms, which also sold eggs to nearby townspeople, the eating of chickens was not frequently done. It tended to be expensive, for its rarity, and it was eaten, generally, on special occasions.

Toward the end of the nineteenth century, farms developed in the United States, which raised broilers; "spring chickens," young male chickens, not needed in the egg industry, which was still the main focus of chicken farming; and "stewing hens," hens which were past their prime in egg laying, for the city markets. Prior to refrigerated trains or trucks, poultry was shipped live, or killed, plucked, and packed on ice, but not eviscerated. Once these chickens arrived in the city, the chickens were cleaned and cut by the neighborhood butcher. Cleaning poultry at home was also still a commonplace practice.

Early in the twentieth century the discovery of vitamin D made possible the productive confinement of chickens year-round. Egg laying chickens could now lay also in the winter, and broilers continued to grow even in the winter. Prior to that discovery, winter was an off season for egg production and meat production. The administration of vitamin D lowered costs, especially for broilers.[93]

Following the administration of vitamin D, production improvements took place which gradually evolved toward factory farms. The major first event was in the 1930s when a Gainesville, Georgia feed salesman named Jesse Jewell offered north Georgia farmers a deal: he would sell them baby chicks and feed on credit. When the chicks were grown, Jewell's company, J. D. Jewell, would buy back the adult chickens (broilers) at a price that would cover his costs and guarantee farmers a profit. Once Jewell signed on enough farmers to produce broilers for him, he invested in his own processing plant and hatchery. Mr. Jewell's company, and others who were starting in this industry, got a large boost during the Second World War,

---

93   http://en.widipedia.org/wiki/Industrial_agriculture%animals%29

1941-1945, when the War Food Administration reserved all processed chicken in north Georgia to prepare meals for troops. This provided J. D. Jewell with a guaranteed purchaser, and permitted the accumulation of capitol for post war development.[94]

CHICKEN FACTORY FARMS

BY MID 1930's, JOHN Tyson in Arkansas, started his business of hauling broilers from local farmers to markets in the north. Ten years later, Tyson, using Jewell's system of contracting, developed an integrated feed and slaughter operation.[95] Thus, the broiler industry started in the South, where it remains, with about 60 companies contracting and supervising individual chicken farmers.[96]

This demonstrates how the factory farm system for chickens is structured. For broilers, there are bout 60 major companies. These possess hatcheries, feed-mills, slaughter houses, and rendering plants. They each contract with individual farmers to raise the chickens to slaughter weight. The individual farmer receives the chicks and the feed, along with its additives, from the company, and the farmer must provide the coops and labor. The companies provide supervisory advice on how to house the chickens, how to debeak them, etc. It is the responsibility of the farmer to raise the chickens with a minimum of mortality and a maximum weight increase, because the farmer gets paid for the total weight of the living chickens delivered to the company. With the cost of the buildings and labor, such contract farming is not very profitable. Should disease or some calamity significantly reduce the flock, the farmer has to absorb the loss. The companies bear no responsibility for the farmer, and contracts are written which vastly benefit the company. The margin of profit is so close, so small, that the farmers readily agree to house the chickens in the most compact manner, thereby limited the space and limiting the amount of labor required.[97] The result is a factory farm.

Egg production differs from broiler production in that egg producing factory farms are distributed nationwide. Broilers, when processed, can

94 The New Georgia Encyclopedia, Poultry, found in http://www. georgiaencyclopedia.org/nge/Article.jsp?id=h-1811

95 http://www.tyson.com/

96 http://www.idausa.org/facts/factoryfarmfacts.html

97 http://www.alabamapoultry.org/beginner.html#intro

be frozen, and sent anywhere from the South. Eggs need to be relatively close to their market. But the same system obtains. Individual farmers are contracted with. The companies guarantee chicks and purchase of all eggs.

The companies also provide supervision for the farmers, and the result is factory farms with far more inhumane treatment of the egg producing chickens. Whereas, the raising of broilers does involve the raising of especially bred chickens with outsized breasts and legs, which limits their ability to move, these chickens, however, do get to survive in larger pens which are less crowded. The concern is not to bruise the breasts or legs. Egg laying chickens, however, are put in small cages called batteries. Within these four to eleven hens are stuffed in a two foot by two foot cage, so small that they can barely move. These battery cages have screened floors, through which most excrement passes. Further, lines of batteries are put upon other batteries, sometimes for several layers. Excrement, therefore, passes on to the backs of the birds below.[98] It is in these battery cages that the hens lay their eggs, which roll out on the forward tilting wire floor, so that they do not get crushed by the other battery inhabitants.

THE CORN DIET

THE FOOD PROVIDED TO these hens, consistent with the logic of all factory farm companies, is primarily of the cheapest grain available, which in the United States, thanks to a generous agricultural subsidy from the United States government, is corn.[99] In 2004 the United States subsidy for feed grains, which are corn, sorghum, oats, and barley[100], accounted for $2,841 million, and 35.4% of all agricultural subsidies. That 2.8 billion dollars did not include soybeans, which received a separate subsidy. Thus, a surfeit of corn is annually produced in the United States, which finds its way as the dominant ingredient in the feed for cattle, swine, and chickens, as well as for many other products, which will be discussed below.

---

98   http://www.wsn.org/factoryfarm/chickenart.html

99   http://en.wikipedia.org/wiki/Compound_feed and http://www.signonsandiego.com/uniontrib/20080323/news_1n23eggs

100   http://en.wikipedia.org/wiki/Compound_feed

The Use of Antibiotics

ANTIBIOTICS HAVE BEEN USED on poultry in poultry factory farms since the 1940's.[101] Since early 2006 four companies controlling most of the chicken factory farms, Tyson Foods, Gold Kist, Perdue Farms, and Foster Farms, have sharply cut back on their use of antibiotics in the feed of chickens that are not sick. The second largest holder of chicken factory farms, Pilgrim's Pride, as of this writing, has declined to cut back their use of antibiotics in chicken feed.[102]

Antibiotics are not usually absorbed by the intestines, leading to the blood stream and taken to the cells generally. Therefore, they do not get into the muscle, which is eaten as meat. Ingested antibiotics, however, do get filtered by the liver. This becomes problematic when a toxin is included in such antibiotic. After 2000 the antibiotic named Roxarsone was introduced and used to protect chickens against disease and to promote growth. Roxarsone contains arsenic. The EPA found that, in chicken liver samples they examined, contained sufficient arsenic to cause neurological problems in a child who ate two ounces of cooked liver per week, or in an adult who ate 5.5 ounces per week. The FDA, with less stringent arsenic standards than the EPA, found no detectable arsenic in their samples of muscle.[103]

But the danger of the evolution of antibiotic resistant pathogens from the widespread use of antibiotics in chicken food remains. Campylobacter (*Campylobacter jejuni*) is a bacterium which lives peacefully in the intestines of chickens. It is a pathogen to people, which causes diarrhea, when people eat undercooked chicken. In 1989, none of the Campylobacter strains, from ill persons, tested by the CDC were resistant to fluoroquinolone antibiotics. In 1995 the FDA approved the use of fluoroquinolones in poultry. Soon after, doctors found Campylobacter strains from ill persons that were resistant to fluoroquinolone antibiotics.[104] By 2000, the FDA

---

101   http://en.wikipedia.org/wiki/Chicken

102   Action Center, "Campaign to End Antibiotic Overuse," in http://actionnetwork. org/stopsuperbugsnow/alert-description.tcl?alert

103   103http://www.consumerreports.org/cro/food/food-safety/animal-feed-and-the-food-supply-105/chicken-arsenic-and-antibiotics/indes.htm

104   From the FAQ section of CDC NARMS Web site: www.ce.gov/narms

banned the use fluoroquinolone use in chickens.[105] But the horse had already left the barn.

The Use of Hormones

Chickens grow much more rapidly than they once did. Some people believe that such growth is the product of hormones; however, farmers had attained rapid growth rates by selective breeding. The use of hormones for chickens has been illegal in the United States since 1959.[106]

> The only hormone that was ever used in any quantity on poultry (DES, [Diethylstilbestrol][107]) was banned in 1959, after everyone but a few die-hard farmers had given them up as a silly idea. Hormones are now illegal in poultry and eggs. The people who advertise "No hormones" are either woefully ignorant or are indulging in cynical fear-mongering, maybe both.[108]

Other Items

People working in or near poultry battery farms are at a health risk.

> The US Department of health released a list of risks to humans working in poultry battery farms and those living nearby, which included respiratory illnesses and musculoskeletal injuries, infections, odors and flies and chemical and infectious compounds in the soil which included the mixtures of antibiotics, pathogens, nutrients, pesticides, hormones and other chemicals are found in or are administered to battery poultry. Trace elements of copper arsenic were also found.[109]

So, we see that the factory farm method of raising boilers or eggs is part of the system of poisoning Americans. These chickens are never outdoors; they do not eat insects or larvae. Their diet is exclusively a mixture of grain and drugs, a major component of which is corn. Thus,

---

105 http://www.cdc.gov/narms/gsf_spotlight/landmarks.pdf

106 http://en.wikipedia.org/wiki/Chicken

107 Diethylstilbestrol is a nonsteroidal estrogen.

108 http://www.plamondon.com/faq_myths.html

109 http://en.wikipedia.org/wiki/Poultry_farming

the meat and eggs are bland and have a surfeit of linoleic acid (omega 6) and exceedingly little alpha-linolenic acid (omega 3). Therefore, as with the beef, these eggs and chicken meat help produce the battery of diseases afflicting adult Americans, as well as the high rate of premature death from disease.

If some demon wanted to arrange for the production of chicken meat and eggs to undermine the health of the American people, he couldn't have done it better than is being done by American chicken factory farmers.

5 - The Production of Pork

PORK IS THE THIRD and last major meat production system we will discuss in this essay. The three meat production systems, beef, chicken, and pork, represent virtually all, if not all, of the intensive, terrestrial industrial type farm operations in this, and other, countries. Included in such systems is the battery system of egg production, which we covered in our discussion of chicken factory farms.

As we have already covered the use of antibiotics in our discussion of beef and chicken production, and hormones in our discussion of beef production, we will not reproduce what has already been said. With respect to the use of corn in swine/pig feed, we will establish that, but not elaborate on it; it has been covered above, and will be discussed again in the next chapter.

THE ORIGIN OF THE DOMESTICATED PIG

THE PIG WAS ONE of the first animals domesticated as livestock for food, leather, and other parts of the animal. It was domesticated just half a century after goats and sheep around 10,500 years ago, in the Near East or/ and in China from the wild boar.[110] The adaptable nature and omnivorous diet of the pig was convenient for people who could feed it food scraps. The pigs also churned up the ground looking for truffles, a fungus, which

---

110 "How the First Farmers Colonized the Mediterranean" The New York Times, August 15, 2008, in http://www.nytimes.com/2008/08/11/science/12visuals. html?ref=science

the people came to appreciate as a food also. The churning of the ground may have also facilitated ploughing.

The pigs were kept mostly for food, but their hides also served for shields and shoes; their bones could be made into tools and needles, and their hairs could serve for brushes.[111]

"Pork" refers to the flesh of a pig, the term coming to us from Middle English, deriving, from the French word, "porc," which derives from the Latin "porcus," meaning pig. Pork is one of the almost 500 French words pertaining to cooking, food or eating that had entered English usage after the Norman Conquest.[112]

PIG FACTORY FARMS

PIG FARMS ARE CONCENTRATED in the United States into a dwindling number. Companies which market 5,000 head or more accounted for 80% of the hog market in 2001. There are about 150 companies which marketed more than 50,000 head annually.[113] The largest such company is Smithfield Foods, Inc., with headquarters in Smithfield, Virginia, and operations in 26 states and 9 countries. It markets 27 million head annually. It produced 5.9 billion pounds of pork in 2006.[114]

Intensive piggeries, or hog lots, are a type of factory farm specialized for the raising of domestic pigs up to slaughter weight. In this system grower pigs are housed indoors in group-housing or straw-lined sheds, while pregnant sows are confined in sow stalls, also known as gestation crates, and give birth in farrowing crates. These gestation crates are barely wider than the sow is, barely longer than she is, and barely taller than she is standing up. The pregnant sow has the choice of standing or squatting down; she can otherwise not move.

The use of these gestation crates for pregnant sows has resulted in lower birth production costs; however, this practice has led to more significant animal welfare concerns. Many of the world's largest producers of pigs, U.S., Canada, Denmark, use gestation crates, but some countries and

---

111   http://en.wikipedia.org/wiki/Pork

112   Bragg, M. The Adventure of English: 500 AD to 2000 (2003), p. 38

113   http://www.engormix.com/swine_production_a_global_e_articles_124_POR.htm

114   http://en.wikipedia.org/wiki/Smithfield_Foods   Smithfield Foods, Inc. also owns and operates beef feedlots, and produced 1.4 billion pounds of beef in 2006.

some states, including the United Kingdom and Florida, California, and Arizona, have banned them.[115]

Pig factory farms, intensive piggeries, are generally large warehouse-like buildings. Indoor pig systems allow the pig's condition to be monitored, ensuring minimum fatalities and increased growth. These buildings are ventilated and their temperature is regulated. Most domestic pig varieties are susceptible to heat stress, and all pigs lack sweat glands and cannot cool themselves. Pigs have a limited tolerance of high temperatures and heat stress can lead to death. Maintaining a more specific temperature within the pig tolerance range also maximized growth and growth to feed ratio.[116] Nevertheless, 6.4% of the pigs die each year from trauma and heat. Respiratory problems and diseases take another 39.1% each year.[117]

THE PIG DIET

THE PIG IS AN omnivore. To ensure growth, grains and legumes are fed to them. The legume most economically available, and fed to them is soybeans. The grain, by virtue of the generous federal subsidy, most economically available, and fed to them is corn. "Although many cereal grains can provide economic sources of energy for pigs in the Midwest, corn is used extensively in Nebraska and South Dakota."[118] This is also true in other states where pig factory farms are. The subsidized corn price makes it relatively cheap throughout the United States.

Because pigs are omnivorous, unlike cattle or chickens, they cannot be harmed or sickened by whatever they are fed, providing it is not toxic, and is nutritious. Pigs are also more particular eaters than chickens or cattle. Changes in a feed mix could cause the pigs to stop eating, at least for a while. This would slow growth, even if just a little. It is very significant to a pig farmer, because her/his margin is evidently smaller than it is for cattle or chicken farms. To make a complete protein, they are given bean meal with their feed, frequently soybean meal. To this meal, corn, or some component or form of corn, is usually mixed in. Corn is the most frequent grain used. So, here is, again, a guarantee that those who eat pork will also get their disproportion of linoleic acid. Although soybeans do have some

---

115   http://en.wikipedia.org/wiki/Intensive_pig_farming

116   *Ibid.*

117   http://www.vivausa.org/campaigns/pigs/report.htm

118   http://www.ianrpubs.unl.edu/epublic/live/ec273/build/ec273.pdf

alpha-linolenic acid, it is not even enough to offset its own linoleic acid. The disproportionate consumption of linoleic acid is also true with factory farmed pork.

THE USE OF ANTIBIOTICS

PIGS ON AMERICAN FACTORY farms are fed a number of antibiotics to control bacteria, as well as a number of other antibiotics to promote growth. The latter do so by also controlling bacteria. The antibiotics which are used are _-lactam antibiotics, including penicillins, lincosamides, and macrolides, including erythromycin and tetracyclines. All of these antibiotics are also used to treat infections in humans.[119]

> Pigs in the USA are exposed to a range of other compounds intended for growth promotion. These include bacitracin, flavophospholipol, pleuromutilins, quinoxalines, virginiamycin and arsenical compounds.[120]

Another antibiotic used in pig factory farms is Carbadox, which is used to promote growth and to prevent dysentery. It is also used against parasite infection. "In early 2004 it was banned by the Canadian government as a livestock feed additive and for human consumption. The European Union also forbids the use of Carbadox at any level. It is approved in the United States for use in swine for up to 42 days before slaughter."[121]

Human health can be affected either by residues of antibiotics in the meat or through the selection of antibiotic resistance which may spread to a human pathogen. The most significant example of the former was the previous use of chloramphenicol, which passed to humans as residues in meat, which coincided with the occurrence of aplastic anaemia in humans. For this reason, as well as the experience of using the drug directly with humans, chloramphenicol was discontinued, and its manufacture in the United States stopped in 1991.

Generally, the residues of antibiotics in meat is insignificant as compared to the spread of antibiotic resistance due to the overuse of antibiotics in

---

119   Hughes, Peter and John Heritage. "Antibiotic Growth-Promoters in Food Animals" in http://www.fao.org/docrep/article/agrippa/555_en.htm

120   http://www.fao.org/docrep/article/agrippa/555_en.htm *Idem.*

121   http://en.wikipedia.org/wiki/Carbadox

factory farm feed. John Heritage, an eminent microbiologist at Leeds University in England and his student, Peter Hughes, have said that such resistance may occur in microbes pathogenic for humans, or it may occur among zoonotic bacteria that subsequently cause disease among humans. Because it is the common occurrence among bacteria to transfer sections of their DNA among each other, another component of this problem would be the development of resistance of a bacterium which is a member of the commensal flora of the animal fed growth promoter. Should this occur, the resistance may transfer to human or animal pathogens.

> Modern medicine has furnished us with a wealth of antibiotics but...alternatives are starting to run out. The four types of bacteria most commonly associated with resistance due to use are *Salmonella, Campylobacter, Escherichia coli* and the enterococci; these bacteria are likely to be transmitted frequently from animals to humans.[122]

In 1999, in a study published in the New England Journal of Medicine, the link between the factory pig farm and resistant Salmonella is solidified. In the reported case the people became ill from eating pork.

> The study describes an outbreak in Denmark of Salmonella DT 104, and especially virulent strain of foodborne disease that causes diarrhea, fever, abdominal cramps, and in some cases death. DT 104 is doubly notorious in the public health community for its resistance to five important antibiotics, including ampicillin and tetracycline.[123]

Reference is to a 1998 outbreak of DT 104 in Denmark. Twenty-one adults and children were identified as having acquired the disease directly or indirectly through contaminated pork. By the time th outbreak was over, 7 had been hospitalized and 1 had died.

---

122   Hughes, Peter and John Heritage. "Antibiotic Growth-Promoters in Food Animals," in http://www.fao.org/docrep/article/agrippa/555_en.htm

123   The Union of Concerned Scientists in their Food and Electronic Digest, which may be found at: http://www.ucsusa.org/food_and_environment/antibiotics_and_food/outbreak-of-a-resistant-foodborne-illness.html

Genetic fingerprinting of the DT 104 bacterium was done and compared with 90 herds (farms) of swine in Denmark. Two herds tested positive; the two farms shared machinery.

This study has severe implications for public health. In addition to DT 104's resistance to five important antibiotics, resistance is also for a group of antibiotics called fluoroquinolones. These are the drugs of first choice for fighting serious salmonella infections.

Doctors in this study reported reduced effectiveness of fluoroquinolone drugs when treating patients during this outbreak. Although it was not possible to directly link the development of resistance in the salmonella to fluoroquinolone use on the swine farms, the practice is a plausible cause. While quinolone drugs had not been used in the two herds that year, the drugs had been used on nearby farms and salmonella is thought to move easily between herds. In Denmark, veterinarians have been licensed to use fluoroquinolones since 1993.

DT 104 has also become a problem in the United States. Reports of reduced effectiveness of the fluoroquinolone drugs against Salmonella DT 104 have increased substantially in the past few years. Outbreaks of the multi-antibiotic-resistant DT 104 strain have recently occurred in California, Vermont, and Washington State. The Centers for Disease Control and Prevention reports that salmonella poisoning (all strains) may affect up 2 million people annually in the United States and about 500 of these die each year.[124]

Another consequence of the frequent and heavy use of antibiotics for pig defense against pathogens as well as for pig growth is the spread of methicillin resistant staphylococcus aureus (MRSA). It is quite true that the first emergence of MRSA was in the 1960's, and derived from the overuse of antibiotics by physicians responding to young mothers and overuse in hospitals. It became a problem, mostly in hospitals, and it affected mostly elderly patients in hospitals.[125] Then in 2003, in the Netherlands, a new strain of MRSA emerged which could not be typed with Sma1 pulsed-field gel electrophoresis,[126] which was then labeled " NT-

---

124   *Idem.*

125   Michael Pollan discusses this in his New York Times essay, "Our Decrepit Food Factories," published on December 16, 2007.

126   "pulsed-field gel electrophoresis" is a method of genotyping specific organisms, and Sma1 was the typed methicillin resistant staphylococcus aureus which was known prior to the discovery in the Netherlands. The process is explained in http://en.wikipedia.org/wiki/Pulsed_field_gel_electrophoresis

MRSA."[127] The conclusion of the analysis of data was that this new strain of MRSA affecting people derived from pig factory farms, and probably, though more data has yet to be collected, from cattle factory farms.

That was 2003, in the Netherlands. On November 6, 2007 Bio-Medicine reported a new study revealing MRSA bacteria in Canadian pig factory farms.[128] The study found NT-MRSA in 45% of the pig farms in Ontario, on which 25% of the pigs carried MRSA, and 20% of the farm workers carried MRSA, a much higher percentage than in the general North American population. The article also mentioned that an estimated nine million hogs were to be imported to the USA that year, 2007.

Although this book focuses on the unhealthy nature of factory farm meat, eggs, and dairy products, we have discussed, as part of what's wrong with factory farms, the wholesale, reckless administration of antibiotics to the farm animals. And, of course, such administration of antibiotics will produce resistant bacteria for most pathogenic bacteria. It is just a matter of time, but it does not take long. The length of time it takes the average bacterium to reproduce is 10 minutes. That converts 1 bacterium to 64 bacteria in one hour, 4,096 in two hours, 262,144 in three hours, and 687,194,476 in four hours. So, they can sustain many casualties, but even if only one survives, the entire complement of pathogens can be reconstituted in a matter of a day, and this time it is resistant.

Of course it foolhardy to use antibiotics non-therapeutically in such a wholesale reckless way. But the factory farms are locked in. If they are going to take the unnatural step of confining the animals to very close quarters, they are created a disease generation system; so, they "have" to use the antibiotics. But this is futile, because the antibiotics only serve to cause the evolution of antibiotic resistant pathogens. This is worse than the unhealthy food. For, if someone becomes aware of how unhealthy the factory farm food is, which they can do by reading this book, and are moved to henceforth only eat healthy food, which is identified also in this book, they can overcome their deficiency disease, and they can become healthy. But if the factory farms generate a number of pathogens resistant

---

127 The investigation and findings are reported in van Loo, Inge; Huijsdens, X; Tiemersma, E; de Neeling, A; vande Sande-Bruinsma, N; Beaujean, D; Voss, A, Kluytmans, J. "Emergence of Methicilin-resistant Staphylococcus aureus of animal origin in humans," Emerging Infectious Diseases, Dec. 2007, found in http://findarticles.com/p/articles/mi_m0GVK/is_12_13/ai_n21168598

128 Article may be found in http://www.bio-medicine.org/ , the title of the article is "New Study Reveals MRSA Bacteria Common Among Pigs and Farm Workers."

to any antibiotic which now exists, then, regardless of what kind of food you eat, you can become a victim of such a pathogen. The human body has not had enough time to evolve immunity to many of the serious disease pathogens, even before they have become resistant. That's why they are called "serious disease pathogens." The ones we have immunity for don't rank. But if we, heretofore, got infected with streptococcus, as an example, a physician could always be assumed to have the medication to handle it. But once this bacterium becomes resistant, physicians may not have an antibiotic which would be effective against it. An effective antibiotic may only be available in the local hospital. But once in the hospital, in this new age of resistant pathogens, there is a strong probability that we would become infected with others.

So, you see that the careless, reckless use of antibiotics by factory farms has endangered the entire population. Therefore, the factory farm use of antibiotics is a far greater injury to the American people, to the people of North America, and to the people of Europe. This injury will cost many lives, ultimately more than from the unhealthy food, and it will persist for a long time.

THE USE OF HORMONES

IN ONTARIO, RESEARCHERS FOUND estrogen, as well as antibiotics, downstream from a factory pig farm.[129] In another study, data gathered from the manure holding pits of 8 dairy farms and 11 swine facilities demonstrated the use of beta-estradiol, alpha-estradiol, and estrone, three sex hormones used in those farms.[130] In addition to estrogen and the related sex hormones listed in the previous sentence, fabricated prostaglandins[131] are given to sows prior to and during pregnancy, and hormones entitled

---

129 Sanderson, H. RA Brain, DJ Johnson, CJ Wilson, and KR Solomon. 2004. Toxicity Classification and Evaluation of Four Pharmaceuticals Classes: Antibiotics, Antineoplastics, Cardiovascular, and Sex Hormones. Toxicology. 203(1-3):27-40.

130 Raman, DR, EL Williams, AC Layton, RT Burns, JP Easter, AS Daugherty, MD Mullen, and GS Sayler. 2004. Estrogen Content of Dairy and Swine Wastes. Environmental Science and Technology. 38(13): 3567-3573.

131 Prostaglandins are signaling molecules which operate in the cells of mammals.

"milk let down products" are given post parturition. Pigs raised for meat are given growth hormones.[132]

We know, already, that factory farms pump hormones in their animals to enhance performance and/or growth. But the inhumanity of doing that is now our concern. As with cattle hormones, the hormones given to pigs find their way into their manure, and then to commercial vegetable farmers. Also, it has been established that these hormones also persist in the downstream fresh water streams, which feed to bigger streams and then to rivers, where they become the drinking water of cities. The water that is not taken in by cities continues downstream, altering and killing fish. It is not only what they do to their animals, it is the damage also done to the ecology, the ecology in which we all live, that is part the of atrocity that is the factory farm.

OTHER ITEMS

IT IS NOT ONLY the eating of factory farm pork, or interacting directly with the animals or the worker that can put you in jeopardy of getting an antibiotic resistant bug, eating commercial vegetables could accomplish the same result.

> Scientists took lettuce, corn, and potatoes and grew them using soil treated with hog manure that had commonly used livestock antibiotic Sulfamethazine in it. All three plants uptook the Sulfamethazine.[133]

---

132   Blayney, Don p.; Fallert, Richard F.; Shagam, Shayle D.; and Ott, Stephen L. "Controversy over livestock growth hormones continues" in http://findarticles.com/p/articles/mi_m3765/is_n4_v14/ai_12619619

133   http://scienceblogs.com/Angrytoxicologist/2007/08/antiobiotic_salad_anyone.php

6 - The Ubiquity of
Corn in the American Diet

THE FEDERAL SUBSIDIZATION OF corn and the tariff against the importation of sugar has created a wide ranging corn based diet, for most livestock as well as for most Americans, thereby creating an over consumption of linoleic acid (Omega 6 fatty acid) and a concomitant over incidence of hypertension, neoplastic cancers, ischemic heart disease, and death, as well as the over incidence of depression. I have already described the widespread use of corn as feed for cattle, chickens, and pigs. Let me now describe the invasive use of corn in human food and pharmaceutical items.

The Iowa Corn Promotion Board lists the varied uses of its corn under five headings: Corn Starches, Corn Syrups, High Fructose Corn Syrups, Dextrose, and Fermentation & Other Chemical Products.[134]

Corn Starches; Food & Drug Uses
- Antibiotics
- Aspirin
- Baked Goods
- Candies
- Condiments
- Mixes & Instant Preparations
- Processed Meats
- Puddings

---

134   "Corn Use & Education," Iowa Corn Promotion Board, found in http://www.iowacorn.org/cornuse_6.html

Corn Syrups; Food & Drug Uses
- Baby Food
- Bologna and Hot Dogs
- Chewing Gum
- Cookies & Crackers
- Dessert Mixes
- Fruit Drinks
- Canned Foods
- Cereals
- Medicinal Syrups
- Pickles
- Salad Dressings
- Seasoning Mixes

High Fructose Corn Syrup
- Carbonated Beverages
- Fruit Fillings
- Cereals
- Frostings
- Ice Cream & Frozen Desserts
- Pancakes
- Pastries
- Relishes & Sauces
- Syrups & Dessert Toppings

Dextrose; Food & Drug Uses
- Antibiotics
- Brownies & Baked Goods
- Canned Fruits
- Cheese Spreads
- Cured Meats (such as bacon)
- Dessert Mixes
- Intravenous Solutions
- Jams & Jellies
- Soda Fountain Preparations
- Marshmallows
- Soups

Fermentation & Other Chemical Products
- Citric Acid
- Lactic Acid
- Essential Amino Acids
- Sugar Alcohols

Using United States Department of Agriculture statistics, the Iowa Corn Promotion Board also published the following national quantitative statistics:[135]

Animal Feed: 5.6 billion bushels of corn went to feed animals. The 510 million bushels of Iowa's corn crop was distributed as follows: 47% went to hogs, 29% to beef cattle, 18% to poultry, and 6% to dairy cattle.

Exports: More than 2.1 billion bushels were exported to other countries.
Corn Sweeteners: 753 million bushels were refined into corn sweeteners. These were used chiefly in colas, candies, cakes and cookies, lunch meats, jams and jellies, snack foods, salad dressing, and ice cream.

Ethanol: 2.1 billion bushels of corn were fermented into fuel alcohol.

Other Uses: 272 million bushels were processed into starch for food and industrial uses: paper, textiles, adhesives, plastics, baked goods, condiments, candies, soups and mixes.

190 million bushels became breakfast cereals, snack chips, tortillas and other corn foods.

137 million bushels of corn were fermented into alcoholic beverages.

Because sweetener, starch, and alcohol production doesn't use all of the corn kernel, the 3.5 billion bushels that went into those products also provided 29.4 million tons of animal feed and 3.3 billion pounds of corn oil.

Now you have an idea of the distribution of corn among foods and drugs of America, and the term "ubiquity" is not inappropriate. One need only go into any commercial grocery store, supermarket, of any city or town of the United States, and look at the ingredients of almost any packaged food item. Also read the ingredients of the dry dog food packages, or of the

---

135   http://www.iowacorn.org/cornuse/documents/
HowisOurCornCropUsed-0607.pdf

dry cat food packages. You will find some form of corn in practically all of them. This means that not only humans, but their pets are consuming a disproportion of linoleic acid (omega 6 fatty acid). So, not only do the pharmacies and physicians get plenty of business mistreating deficiency diseases in people, but the veterinarians get to examine and prescribe veterinary prescriptions for the "mysterious" emergence of hepatitis in middle aged dogs, another deficiency disease. So, not only do we have the highest rate of disease among our people, in the world, but we probably also have the most diseased dogs, as well as cats.[136]

Let us now review the casualty figures for being subjected to this corn diet. Unbalanced, disproportionate linoleic acid (omega 6 fatty acid) from the over consumption, and for many Americans, unwitting over consumption, of corn results in hypertension for an increasing number of Americans, which afflicts 25% of all adult Americans, and the percentage increases with age, the older Americans having over consumed corn for more time.[137] Chronic hypertension leads to ischemic heart disease, which culminates in a heart attack. The United States not only has the highest rate of hypertension, but also highest rate of annual coronary heart attack deaths. 400,000 die each year of coronary heart attacks.[138]

The disproportionate distribution of arachidonic acid, in each of the 100 billion[139] cells of the human body, also tends to form neoplasms, tumors. This is also known as cancer, and it is difficult to get a figure on the incidence of cancerous tumors afflicting Americans. But the particular neoplasm referred to as breast cancer does have incidence figures. Thus we know that there are 180,000 women afflicted with breast cancer annually.[140]

---

136   Open confession: This author only has dogs as pets; he has no direct knowledge of cats.

137   From the National Heart, Lung, and Blood Institute website at http://www.nhlbi.nih.gov/hbp/intro.htm

138   http://en.wikipedia.org/wiki/Heart_attacks

139   It seems that nobody has sat down and counted the cells in the average human body. Estimates go from 10 billion to 100 trillion. And there are the same number, if not more, commensal bacteria in the human body. So, without taking any number seriously, let us agree that there are a great number of cells and organisms in the human body.

140   Rose DP and Connolly JM. "Effects of dietary omega-3 fatty acids on human breast cancer growth and metastases in nude mice," National Cancer Institute 1993 Nov 3;85(21):1743-7 retrieved in http://www.ncbi.nlm.nhih.gov/pubmed/8411258

Although it is a much smaller number, we do not have the number of males afflicted with breast cancer.

In addition to causing neoplasms the disproportionate distribution of arachidonic acid in each of the 100 billion cells of the human body from the over consumption of corn also interferes with the immune system, causing autoimmune disorders. This produced a number of deficiency diseases. Perhaps the most common is rheumatoid arthritis, which afflicts about 200,000 persons annually.[141] There is also the deficiency autoimmune condition of hypersensitivity, which are differentiated into anaphylaxis, cytotoxis, and immune complex disease. We have no figures for these. Another autoimmune disorder which may be related to deficiency of omega 3 fatty acids is Celiac Disease. It afflicts 1 in 250 for an estimated condition. One in 4,700 have been diagnosed with the condition.

When arachidonic acid is disproportionately distributed in the brain, where the acid normally is, it causes depression and possibly schizophrenia. Between 13% and 27% of all American adults are estimated to have sub-clinical depression.[142] An estimated 2.2 million Americans are afflicted with schizophrenia.[143]

Finally, and only indirectly related to the corn diet, and directly related to the irresponsible operation of factory farms, 300,000 Americans are hospitalized each year because of food-borne illnesses, and 5,000 of these die each year.

So, there we are. The over consumption of corn is responsible for almost 80 million Americans suffering from deficiency disease, which is also responsible for about 400,000 coronary deaths each year. For perspective, the corn death toll is equivalent to 167 September 11, 2001 deaths. In response to the terrorist attack on U.S. soil, killing almost 3,000 innocents, the President dispatched the armed forces overseas. It seems to me that if you have factory farms causing 167 times the death toll each year, it would warrant the dispatch of the armed forces, or some other force, to end this scourge on the American people.

But let us dispassionately investigate the cause of all this? As with any major human problem, the causes are numerous. However, we can identify the base causes, and these are: ignorance, shortsightedness, greed, and

---

141   http://en.wikipedia.org/wiki/Rheumatodid_arthritis http://en.wikipedia.org/wiki/Rheumatodid_arthritis The 1% is applied against an assumed adult U.S. population of 200,000,000.

142   http://www.wrongdiagnoses.com/d/depression/prevalence.htm

143   http://www.schizophrenia.com/szfacts.htm

irresponsibility. It is quit possible that the farmers and the owners of the factory farms are unaware of the consequences of an almost exclusive corn diet, and of the need for humans to receive both omega 6 fatty acids and omega 3 fatty acids in close proportion. If so, it will be the responsibility of public authority to act to protect the public's health. And, in this respect, it seems that Congress should be assumed to be aware of the need for a balanced diet of fatty acids, and of the severe consequences of ill health from an almost exclusive corn diet. Even if Congressmen are not aware of these facts, their staffs should be assumed to be so aware. The findings about the function of the essential fatty acids have been published for well over ten years, and several books on the subject have been published. Perhaps they have not taken advantage of this knowledge, and are still ignorant. But the same cannot be said for the United States Public Health Service, the Surgeon General, who is the ranking officer of that service, nor the Assistant Secretary of Health, to whom the Surgeon General answers, and who is the principal advisor to the Secretary of Health and Human Services (DHHS)[144] on public health and scientific issues. These people must be assumed to understand the deleterious consequences of feeding all food livestock in factory farms corn, and inserting corn or corn products in most packaged foods in commercial supermarkets. The Surgeon General's particular authority is to educate the public about major public health issues.[145] A system which sickens 80 million Americans and causes the annual death of more than 400,000 certainly is a major public issue. What educational campaign has the Surgeon General launched on this issue? None, none whatsoever. The Assistant Secretary of Health must be presumed to be aware. The Assistant Secretary of Health is supposed to advise the Secretary of DHHS on major public health issues. And the Assistant Secretary of Health can also prepare proposed legislation to deal with a major public health issue. Is there any evidence that the DHHS has acted in any way on this issue? None, none whatsoever.

There is the United States Department of Agriculture Food Safety and Inspection Service, (USDAFSIS) which is responsible for inspecting meats for safety. We have established that the beef from corn fed feedlot cattle, and the meat and eggs from corn fed chicken factory farms, and the pork from corn fed pig factory farms is unsafe and dangerous to consumers' health to the extent that we may consider such meats as poisons. Yet the

---

144   http://en.wikipedia.org/wiki/U.S._Department_of_Health_and_Human_Services

145   http://en.wikipedia.org/wiki/U.S._Surgeon_General

factory farms call the meat "food," and it is distributed in supermarkets as "food." What regulations has the USDAFSIS issued to deal with these dangerous meats? None, none whatsoever. Well, there is still the Food and Drug Administration. The agency is responsible for the safety of cosmetics,[146] and we have seen that many of the body and hand creams, which penetrate the skin, contain corn products, thereby delivering a disproportionate amount of linoleic acid (omega 6 fatty acid) to the user's system. These are dangerous and unhealthy products. What has the FDA done about them? Nothing, absolutely nothing.

Seventy percent of all antibiotics are distributed by the CAFOs. It is clear who is responsible for the evolution of campylobacter, Salmonella, and NT-MRSA of the antibiotic resistant bacteria. And the FDA has done nothing. Nothing, absolutely nothing..

So the Federal Government is batting zero in this major health crisis of America. Actually, our federal system is batting less than zero, because Congress, in its wisdom, has passed laws, administered by the Department of Agriculture, which subsidize the growing of corn. It also, in its respect for international free trade, has erected high tariffs against the importation of cane sugar. So, now you can understand why corn sweeteners are universal in this country. Corn sweeteners, such as High Fructose Corn Syrup, have fructose as their sweetening agent. Fructose is not as easily digested as sucrose, and the body's use of it is less efficient. Corn sweeteners are also not preferred by major users. Coca Cola, for instance, uses cane sugar in its beverages bottled in other countries. In the United States, bowing to strong economic logic, it uses corn sweetener.

The FDA has also demonstrated its commitment, not to health and safety, but to poor health and, ultimately, disease. In 2004 Paramount Farms, a large factory almond farm in California, which bares the earth beneath the trees with strong herbicides and which, probably, fertilized the trees with disease infested manure from factory animal farms, was found to have its raw almonds infested with Salmonella Enteriditis.[147] In response, acting evidently on the advise of Paramount Farms, the FDA required the pasteurization of all Paramount Farms almonds, as well as of all almonds of all other farms. This was done although there was no evidence of any Salmonella, or any other infestation in the raw almonds of any of the organic almond farms. Further, the FDA stipulated that the manner of pasteurization has to be one of the following three methods:

146   http://en.wikipedia.org/wiki/FDA

147   http://www.fda.gov/oc/po/firmrecalls/almonds.html

- Fumigation with propylene oxide, a known carcinogen.[148]
- High Heat, which degrades the integrity of the nuts and enzyme structure.
- Steam Pasteurization, which degrades nutrients, enzymes, and antioxidants.

So, here is the FDA unnecessarily reducing the nutrition of almonds by processing them, and allowing one method to be used with is downright unhealthy, prone to result in cancer. Further, the FDA, in a transparently fraudulent act, is requiring that these processed almonds be marketed as "raw almonds." So much for the federal government acting on behalf of its citizens.

It is quite apparent that the U.S. government is not even neutral in this national crisis. In the last analysis, in the face of the impotence of the government to respond to this massive health problem, it is Congress, the representative of the people, which has the responsibility to act to end this health disaster. But instead, what is this great democratic institution, the representative of the people, doing? It is enabling this program with massive subsidies for corn, which sickens and kills hundreds of thousands of Americans each year. And we're paying for it.

Since public authority is no help, we will have to act on our own. There are ways to avoid the over consumption of corn, and eat a healthy diet.

---

148 http://www.rense.com/general77/almonds.htm

7 - The Healthy Diet

A HEALTHY DIET IS the eating of uncontaminated food, which contains all of the essential vitamins, fatty acids, minerals, and fiber. Following is a detailed discussion of these requisites.

There are 13 vitamins essential for human health. Vitamin D is made when a human's skin is exposed to the ultraviolet rays of the sun. It is also available from certain foods, mainly animal products and whole grain cereals. People in northern latitudes have to also supplement Vitamin D in pill form for them to get the adequate daily amount. The other twelve must be attained by eating certain foods. There are tentative findings about biotin (Vitamin B_7) and pantothenic acid (Vitamin B_5) that the human system can make these vitamins through the agency of its intestinal bacteria, specifically those which colonize the colon. These bacteria, as well as many bacteria in the outside world, can form biotin and pantothenic acid.[149] The tentative findings are that these substances, biotin and pantothenic acid, are passed to the intestinal lining, where the blood stream can absorb them. It is also not yet known whether a significant amount of these two substances are transferred to the blood stream in this way. It is known that Vitamin K is made by the intestinal bacteria.

Below are listed the vitamins by the alphanumeric order, a brief discussion of the importance of each, and the food sources for each, after which the dietary minerals will be discussed.

---

149   The Linus Pauling Institute, from http://lpi.oregonstate.edu/infocenter/vitamins/pa/

THE VITAMINS

Vitamin A – Retinol

Retinol, the animal form of Vitamin A, is a fat soluble vitamin important in vision and bone growth. From animal sources, liver or eggs, retinyl esters are acquired, which can be directly converted to retinol. From plant sources, carrots, spinach, or others listed below, carotenoids are acquired. They go through a two-step process in the body to form retinol and retinoic acid. Retinoic acid is known to affect the differentiation of stem cell to a committed fate. The retina is patterned by retinoic acid.[150] It may not play an active role after embryology. Following are the best food sources for Vitamin A:

- carrots
- broccoli leaves (not broccoli florets)
- sweet potatoes
- kale
- apricots
- spinach
- okra
- onions
- collards
- peaches
- apricots
- papaya
- mustard greens
- peas
- winter squash
- plantains

Vitamin B$_1$ – Thiamin[151]

THIAMIN, ANEURINE HYDROCHLORIDE, IS Vitamin B$_1$, and, as are all of the B vitamins, is water soluble. Thiamin is essential for neural function and carbohydrate metabolism. A severe deficiency in thiamin results in Beriberi, a nerve and heart disease. Following are the best food sources for Vitamin B$_1$:

---

150   From http://en.wikipedia.org/wiki/Retinol

151   This list is derived from USDA National Nutrient Database for Standard Reference, Release 18 http://www/ars.usda.gov/services/docs.htm?docid=9673

- beans, black (turtle)
- beans, navy (white)
- beef, meats and by-products, liver
- beet greens
- beets
- duck
- carrots
- chicken
- buckwheat flour
- rye bread
- cereal, whole wheat farina
- dandelion greens
- peas
- oat bran
- soy beans

Vitamin B$_2$ – Riboflavin[152]

Riboflavin, Vitamin B$_2$, is made up of two enzymes. These are flavin mononucleotide (FMN) and flavin adenine dinucleotide (FAD), which are important in energy production. These coenzymes work as catalysts in the electron transport system, which result in the formation of the primary energy currency in the cell, ATP (adenosine triphosphate). Thus, the ultimate product is energy. Riboflavin is also required for activation and support of activity of Vitamin B$_9$, folate, and Vitamin B$_3$, niacin, and Vitamin K. Following are the best food sources for Vitamin B$_2$:

- turkey
- almonds
- soy nuts
- yogurt
- mushrooms
- avocado
- collard greens
- egg
- soy beans

---

152   The list is combined from http://www.feinberg.northwestern.edu/nutrition/ factsheets/vitamin-b2. html, http://www.trekfit.com/nc/nf_05_b2.html, and http:// www/ars.usda.gov/services/docs.htm?docid=9673

- asparagus
- broccoli

Vitamin B$_3$ – Niacin[153]

Niacin, Vitamin B$_3$, a water soluble vitamin, is also known as nicotinic acid. Nicotinamide is a derivative of nicotinic acid, and is used by the body to form two coenzymes, nicotinamide adenine dinucleotide (NAD) and nicotinamide adenine dinucleotide phosphate (NADP). Although these enzymatic and acidic names are similar, they are not related to the nicotine in tobacco.

Living organisms derive most of their energy from oxidation-reduction (redox) reactions, which are processes involving the transfer of electrons. As many as 200 enzymes require the niacin coenzymes, NAD and NADP, mainly to accept or donate electrons for redox reactions. NAD functions most often in energy producing reactions involving the degradation (catabolism) of carbohydrates, fats, proteins, and alcohol. NADP functions more often in biosynthetic (anabolic) reactions, such as in the synthesis of all macromolecules, including fatty acids and cholesterol. Following are the best food sources for Vitamin B$_3$:

- chicken
- tuna fish
- beef
- fish, halibut
- barley
- bulgur
- mushrooms
- duck

Vitamin B$_5$ – Pantothenic acid[154]

PANTOTHENIC ACID IS WATER soluble Vitamin B$_5$ and is essential to all forms of life. Pantothenic acid is found throughout living cells in the form of coenzyme A (CoA), an essential coenzyme in a variety of reactions that sustain life. CoA is required for chemical reactions that generate energy from food (carbohydrates, proteins, and fats). The synthesis of essential

---

153 This list is derived from USDA National Nutrient Database for Standard Reference, Release 18 http://www/ars.usda.gov/services/docs.htm?docid=9673

154 This list is derived from USDA National Nutrient Database for Standard Reference, Release 18 http://www/ars.usda.gov/services/docs.htm?docid=9673

fats, cholesterol, and steroid hormones requires CoA, as does the synthesis of the neurotransmitter acetylcholine and the hormone melatonin. Heme, a component of hemoglobin, requires a CoA-containing compound for its synthesis. Metabolism of a number of drugs and toxins by the liver requires CoA. Following are the best food sources for Vitamin B_5:

- beef
- mushrooms, shiitake
- chicken
- turkey
- seeds, sunflower
- yogurt
- couscous
- rice, brown or white, long grained
- bulgur
- oat bran
- grapefruit
- potato
- peas

Vitamin B_6 – Pyridoxal 5'-Phosphate [155]

Vitamin B_6 is a water soluble vitamin, which has three forms. Pyridoxal 5'-Phosphate (PLP) is the form most important in human metabolism. PLP, a coenzyme, plays a vital role in the function of approximately 100 enzymes that catalyze essential chemical reactions in the human body. PLP functions as a coenzyme for glycogen phosphorylase, and enzyme that catalyzed the release of glucose from stored glycogen. Much of the PLP in the human body is found in muscles, and bound to glycogen phosphorylase. PLA is also a coenzyme for reactions used to generate glucose from amino acids, a process know as gluconeogenesis. Following are the best food sources for Vitamin B_6:

- fish, tuna
- beef
- turkey
- rice, brown or white, long grained
- potato

---

155   This list is derived from USDA National Nutrient Database for Standard Reference, Release 18 http://www/ars.usda.gov/services/docs.htm?docid=9673

- banana
- plums, prunes
- plantains
- barley
- carrots

Vitamin B$_7$ – Biotin[156]

Biotin is a water soluble vitamin that is attached at the active site of four important enzymes known as carboxylases. 1) Acetyl-CoA carboxylase catalyzes the binding of bicarbonate to acetyl-CoA to form malonyl-CoA. Malonyl-CoA is required for the catalysis of fatty acids. 2) Pyruvate carboxylase is a critical enzyme in gluconeogenesis, the formation of glucose from sources other than carbohydrates, rather from amino acids and fats. 3) Methylcrotonyl-CoA carboxylase catalyzes an essential step in the metabolism of leucine, an essential amino acid. 4) Propionyl-CoA carboxylase catalyzes essential steps in the metabolism of amino acids, cholesterol, and odd chain fatty acids (fatty acids with an odd number of carbon molecules). Following are the best food sources for Vitamin B$_7$:

- peanuts
- hazelnuts
- almonds
- liver
- cheese, Camembert
- yeast, bakers active
- wheat bran, crude
- cashews
- egg
- yogurt
- avocado

---

156   The list for biotin is from the Northwestern University School of Medicine and The Linus Pauling Institute, at http://www.feinberg.northwestern.edu/nutrition/factsheets/biotin.htm and http://lpi.oregonstate.edu/infocenter/vitamins/biotin/ respectively.

Vitamin B$_9$ – Folic acid[157]

VITAMIN B$_9$ IS A water soluble member of the B complex vitamins. In capsule form and in the form of the fortification of fortified foods, the stable form of folic acid is used. In foods where it naturally occurs, it is usually in the form of its anion[158], folate. In its anion form, folate, in collaboration with Vitamins B$_6$ and B$_{12}$, participates in the metabolism of several important amino acids, and in the synthesis of DNA. The latter is particularly important in the gestation of a foetus. It is not uncommon for women, in the midst of a pregnancy, to suffer anemia because of the deficiency of folate in their systems. Following are the best food sources for Vitamin B$_9$:

- rice
- turkey
- black eyed peas
- lentils
- chicken
- pinto beans
- okra
- chick peas (garbanzos)
- spinach
- black (turtle) beans
- soy beans
- collards
- broccoli
- turnip greens

Vitamin B$_{12}$ – Cyanocobalamin[159]

VITAMIN B$_{12}$ IS A water soluble member of the B complex vitamins. It also has the largest and most complex chemical structure of any vitamin. It is also unique among vitamins in that it contains a metal ion, cobalt. For this reason cobalamin is the term used to refer to compounds having Vitamin B$_{12}$ activity. Methylcobalamin and 5-deoxyadenosyl are the forms of

---

157   This list is derived from USDA National Nutrient Database for Standard Reference, Release 18 http://www/ars.usda.gov/services/docs.htm?docid=9673

158   An 'anion' is a negatively charged ion. A positively charged ion is referred to as a 'cation.'

159   This list is derived from USDA National Nutrient Database for Standard Reference, Release 18 http://www/ars.usda.gov/services/docs.htm?docid=9673

Vitamin B_{12} used in the human body. The form of cobalamin used in most supplements, cyanocobalamin, is readily converted to 5-deoxyadenosyl and methylcobalamin in the body. In collaboration with Vitamins B_6 and B_9 Vitamin B_{12} is instrumental in the synthesis of amino acids and of DNA. Following are the best food sources for Vitamin B_{12}:

- clams
- beef
- mollusks, oyster
- chicken
- salmon
- sardine
- herring
- cottage cheese
- turkey
- yogurt

Vitamin C – Ascorbic acid[160]

Vitamin C, which is ascorbic acid, is water soluble, and it is a very effective antioxidant. Unlike most mammals, however, humans do not have the ability to make their own Vitamin C. It must, therefore, be acquired through diet.

Of what is known of Vitamin C, its three major functions are: 1) the synthesis of collagen, an important structural component of blood vessels, tendons, ligaments, and bone; 2) the synthesis of norepinephrine, a neurotransmitter critical to brain function, and is know to affect mood; and 3) the synthesis of carniture, a small molecule essential for the transport of fat to mitochondria, for conversion to energy. Recent research has suggested that Vitamin C is also involved in the metabolism of cholesterol, implying that it maintains low, or reduces, blood cholesterol levels. Following are the best food sources for Vitamin C:

- sweet red pepper
- strawberries
- orange juice
- cranberries
- kohlrabi

---

160   This list is derived from USDA National Nutrient Database for Standard Reference, Release 18 http://www/ars.usda.gov/services/docs.htm?docid=9673

- broccoli
- peas
- potato
- brussels sprouts
- kiwi fruit

Vitamin D – Cholecalciferol[161]

Vitamin D is a fat soluble vitamin that is essential for maintaining normal calcium metabolism. Vitamin D has five forms, Vitamin D_1 through Vitamin D_5. Vitamin D_3 is made and used by humans. Vitamins D_4 and D_5 are derived from Vitamin D_3. Vitamin D_3 is made in the skin when 7-dehydrocholesterol reacts with ultraviolet light at wavelengths between 270 - 300 nm, with peak synthesis occurring between 295 - 297 nm. These wavelengths are present in sunlight at sea level when the sun is more than 45° above the horizon. At this elevation, which occurs daily in the tropics, daily during the spring and summer seasons in temperate regions, and almost never within the arctic and antarctic circles, adequate amounts of Vitamin D_3 can be made in the skin after only ten to fifteen minutes of sun exposure at least two times per week to the face, arms, hands, or back without sunscreen.

The other sources of Vitamin D_3 are from oceanic fish or from supplemental tablets. In the temperate climatic zone, and especially in the norther temperate zone, adequate Vitamin D_3 can be maintained by taking D_3 tablets rated at 1,000 IU, daily. Alternately, one can gain an adequate supply by eating adequate amounts of the following foods daily:

- pink salmon
- mushrooms
- yeast
- rainbow trout
- soy milk, fortified with Vitamin D
- cow's milk, fortified with Vitamin D
- orange juice, fortified with Vitamin D
- cereal, fortified

---

161   Dietary Reference Intakes for Vitamin D http://www.iom.edu/Reports/2010/Dietary-Reference-Intakes-for-Calcium-and-Vitamin-D.aspx

Vitamin E – Tocopherol[162]

Vitamin E is the collective name for a set of eight related tocopherols and tocotrienols, which are fat soluble vitamins with antioxidant properties. Of the eight, alpha-tocopherol has been most studied. Alpha-tocopherol can modulate the inflammatory responses in white blood cells. It can decrease blood clotting by platelets. Alpha-tocopherol also regulates vascular tone, referring to the flexibility of blood vessels.

Very few studies have been done of the role of gamma-tocopherol in the human body, but those that have suggest that it may have potent physiological actions. Both alpha- and gamma-tocopherol are antioxidants, but gamma-tocopherol seems to have an additional, unique, function. "Because of its different chemical structure, gamma-tocopherol scavenges reactive nitrogen species, which, like reactive oxygen species, can damage proteins, lipids, and DNA."[163] Following are the best food sources for Vitamin E:

- tomatoes
- sunflower seeds
- almonds
- hazelnuts
- peanuts
- spinach
- asparagus
- soy milk

Vitamin K – Phylloquinone[164]

Vitamin K is fat soluble. Vitamin K has two forms, K_1 and K_2. K_1 is phylloquinone. It is essential for the functioning of several proteins involved in blood clotting. Plants synthesize phylloquinone, the major of the two forms of Vitamin K, K_1. K_2 is menaquinone, and is normally produced by the intestinal bacteria[165]. The following plants are the main sources of phylloquinone:

162 This list is derived from USDA National Nutrient Database for Standard Reference, Release 18 http://www/ars.usda.gov/services/docs.htm?docid=9673

163 This quote, and much of this narrative, derives from http://lpi.oregonstate.edu/ss03/vitamin.html

164 Sources of food for Vitamin K are derived from The Linus Pauling Institute, at http://lpi.oregonstate.edu/infocenter/vitamins/vitaminK/

165 http://en.wikipedia.org/wiki/Vitamin_K

- kale
- collards
- spinach
- turnip greens
- beet greens
- brussels sprouts
- onions, scallions
- dandelion greens
- parsley
- okra
- cabbage

DIETARY MINERALS

THOSE ELEMENTS WHICH ARE referred to as the essential minerals for healthy functioning of the human body are chemical elements other than carbon, hydrogen, nitrogen, and oxygen and which are present in organic molecules. The essential elements involved in our structure and metabolism are:[166]

Calcium – For muscle, heart and digestive system health, builds bone, neutralized acidity, supports synthesis and function of blood cells.

Chloride – For production of hydrochloric acid in the stomach and in cellular pump functions.

Magnesium – Required for the processing of ATP (Adenosine TriPhosphate) and related reactions; it builds bone and increases alkalinity; it also activates enzymes to metabolize blood sugars, proteins, and carbohydrates.

Phosphorus – Most phosphorus is found in the bone, usually at a 1:2 ratio to calcium. Posphorus is a component of each human cell membrane. Phosphate bonds of ATP provide the energy necessary for metabolism.

---

166 The descriptions of the functions of the essential elements are drawn largely from http://en.wikipedia.org/wiki/Dietary_minerals and http://www.bodyandfitness.com/Information/Health/Research/minerals

Potassium – Potassium is a systemic electrolyte and is essential in coregulating ATP with sodium. Potassium is critical to the transmission of nerve impulses, muscle contractions, and the maintenance of normal blood pressure.

Sodium – Sodium is a system electrolyte, and is essential in coregulating ATP with potassium. Sodium, potassium, and chloride are all necessary for the transmission of electrical impulses between nerve cells.

Zinc – Zinc supports the health of the immune system, normal synthesis of protein, and the health of the reproductive organs, especially in men.

There are a number of minerals required in trace amounts (RDA <200 mg/day). Some are listed alphabetically.

Chromium – Chromium functions as part of several enzyme system, including the glucose tolerance factor, which works with in the utilization of glucose. Chromium is also involved in the metabolism of triglycerides.

Cobalt – Cobalt is the core component of Vitamin B_{12}, which in collaboration with Vitamins B_6 and B_9, is instrumental in the synthesis of amino acids and of DNA.

Copper – Copper is enzymatically involved with the mitochondrion or mitochondria in each cell, in the process of synthesizing ATP.

Iodine – Iodine is essential in the development and functioning of the thyroid gland.

Iron – Iron is required for many proteins and enzymes, notably hemoglobin.

Manganese – Manganese enzymatically dismantles superoxides, negatively charged oxygen radicals, into oxygen and hydrogen peroxide, thereby playing an important antioxidant role. Manganese also is involved in normal bone metabolism.

Molybdenum – Molybdenum is involved with the formation of nucleic acid, thereby assisting in the formation and maintenance of DNA, RNA, and ATP.

Selenium – Selenium is required for antioxidase proteins.

Sulfur – Sulfur, as thiolate, functions as part of the amino acid cysteine, which plays a role in many biological systems. Sulfur also is part of methionine, an alpha-amino acid, an essential amino acid which helps synthesize lecithin and phospholipids, the cell and organelle membranes.

All of these minerals are elements in the Earth's crust. Animals, including humans, cannot use them in their simple elemental form. Plants can take the simple elements and transform them into compound molecules, which humans, and other animals, can use. Therefore, it is necessary for humans to eat the plant sources of these mineral compounds. Alternately, we can eat animals which eat the plants.

Following are the food sources of each mineral:

Calcium[167]
- milk
- cheese, ricotta
- yogurt
- collards
- rhubarb
- fish, sardine
- potato
- tofu
- beans, white (navy), black
- garbanzos
- tahini
- almonds

---

167 This list is derived from USDA National Nutrient Database for Standard Reference, Release 18 http://www/ars.usda.gov/services/docs.htm?docid=9673

- sardines
- salmon
- smelt
- oats
- turnip greens
- bok choy
- okra
- mustard greens
- kale
- beet greens
- turnip greens
- soy beans
- dandelion greens
- navy beans
- black eyed peas
- cheese, Swiss, provolone, cheddar

Chloride[168]

- table salt
- sea salt
- seaweed
- rye
- tomatoes
- lettuce
- celery
- olives

Magnesium[169]

- bulgur
- oat bran
- fish, halibut
- spinach
- barley
- seeds, pumpkin and squash
- soy beans

---

168 The chloride sources are derived from http://www.nim.nih.gov/medlineplus/print/ency/article/002417.htm

169 This list is derived from USDA National Nutrient Database for Standard Reference, Release 18 http://www.ars.usda.gov/services/docs.htm?docid=9673

- navy beans
- black (turtle) beans
- lima beans
- tomato
- Brazil nuts
- artichokes
- beet greens

Phosphorus[170]

- milk
- oat bran*
- barley*
- yogurt
- cheese, ricotta, cottage
- soy beans
- bulgur*
- chickpeas (garbanzos)
- turkey
- fish, halibut, flat fish, haddock, sardine, and salmon
- couscous*
- seeds, sunflower*
- great northern beans
- peanuts*
- lentils*

* Phosphorus from nuts, seeds, and grains is about 50% less bioavailable than phosphorus from other sources, due to the presence of phytic acid in nuts, seeds, and grains. Cooking reduces phytic acid, and the ingestion of the bacteria lactobacillus acidophilus and lactobacillus casei, which are two of the four bacteria used to make yogurt, neutralizes phytic acid. These bacteria, l.acidophilus and l.casei, normally do inhabit the human, and animal, body, and are resident in the intestines, mouth, and vagina. However, this colony may have to be augmented to neutralize the phytic acid of a significant portion of grains, nuts, and seeds. Yogurt can serve to neutralize the phytic acid.

---

170   This list is derived from USDA National Nutrient Database for Standard Reference, Release 18 http://www/ars.usda.gov/services/docs.htm?docid=9673

Potassium[171]

- sweet potato
- beet greens
- white potato
- white beans
- yogurt
- clams
- blackstrap molasses
- fish, halibut
- soybeans, green
- tuna
- lima beans
- winter squash
- fish, rockfish
- fish, cod
- banana
- spinach
- tomato
- peaches
- pork loin
- apricots
- rainbow trout
- cantaloupe
- lentils

Sodium

Sodium occurs naturally in most foods, most commonly in the form of sodium chloride, salt. Quick breads made with baking powder or baking soda have sodium, as do many processed foods. Otherwise, in addition to the minute quantities in drinking water, the following foods naturally have an appreciable amount:

- salt
- miso
- sauerkraut
- soy sauce
- kidney beans

---

171   http://www.health.gov/DIETARYGUIDELINES/dga2005/document/

Zinc[172]

- oysters
- crab, Dungeness
- beef
- pork
- chicken, dark meat
- turkey, dark meat
- duck
- lamb
- barley

Chromium[173]

- broccoli
- green beans
- potatoes
- grape juice
- orange juice
- beef
- turkey breast
- turkey ham
- waffle
- bagel
- apple
- banana

Copper[174]

- beef
- oysters
- lobster
- mushroom, shiitake
- cashews

---

172   This list is derived from USDA National Nutrient Database for Standard Reference, Release 18 http://www/ars.usda.gov/services/docs.htm?docid=9673

173   Http://en.wikipedia.org/wiki/Dietary_Reference_Intake   and   http://lpi.oregonstate.edu/infocenter/minerals/chromium/index.html

174   This list is derived from USDA National Nutrient Database for Standard Reference, Release 18 http://www/ars.usda.gov/services/docs.htm?docid=9673

- soy beans
- barley
- tomato

Iodine[175]

- cod
- shrimp
- sardine
- tuna, canned in oil
- cow's milk
- egg
- navy beans
- potato, w/peel
- turkey breast
- seaweed

Iron[176]

- mollusks, clams and oysters
- turkey
- cereal, whole wheat farina
- chicken
- soy beans
- lentils
- spinach
- duck
- beef, beef liver
- kidney beans
- Jerusalem artichoke
- oat bran
- barley
- chickpeas (garbanzos)
- lima beans
- black eyed peas
- navy beans
- great northern beans
- black (turtle) beans

---

175   http://lpi.oregonstate.edu/infocenter/minerals/iodine/index.html

176   This list is derived from USDA National Nutrient Database for Standard Reference, Release 18 http://www/ars.usda.gov/services/docs.htm?docid=9673

- tomato
- cherries

Manganese[177]

- oat bran
- bulgur
- pineapple
- barley
- spaghetti, whole wheat
- okra
- hazel nuts
- brown rice
- spinach
- chickpeas (garbanzos)
- lima beans
- raspberries

Molybdenum[178]

- beans
- lentils
- peas
- bread, whole wheat
- bread, rye
- oat cereal
- almonds
- walnuts
- cashews

Nickel[179]

- oatmeal
- beans
- peas
- nuts

---

177 This list is derived from USDA National Nutrient Database for Standard Reference, Release 18 http://www/ars.usda.gov/services/docs.htm?docid=9673

178 http://en.wikipedia.org/wiki/Dietary_Reference_Intake and http://lpi.oregonstate.edu/infocenter/minerals/molybdenum/index.html

179 http://jn.nutrition.org/nutinfo/content/nick.shtml and http://www.eco-usa.net/toxics/nickel.shtml

- chocolate
- water

Selenium[180]

- Brazil nuts
- chicken
- fish, tuna, roughy, halibut, rockfish, and salmon
- couscous
- oat bran

Sulfur[181]

- kale
- cabbage
- cauliflower
- horseradish
- cranberries
- meat
- fish
- egg yolks
- onion
- garlic

The food sources for each vitamin and mineral has now been presented. Table 4 presents a consolidated list of all of the foods for all of the vitamins and dietary minerals. Table 5, following, inverts the information in Table 4, and shows which foods correspond to which vitamins and minerals. Only listed in these two tables are the major sources of the vitamins and minerals associated with each food. Many foods have traces of several vitamins and minerals, but only the major sources are listed. As may be seen, this food source list accommodates vegans as well as ovo-vegetarians, ovo-lacto-vegetarians, and omnivores. Vitamin B_{12} can only be made by the bacterial colonies of specific animals. Therefore, it is only available by eating the animals or their products. Vegans, therefore, will have to take vitamin B_{12} from tablets containing it. As dietary minerals must all be moleculized by plants, the mineral food lists, as well as this consolidated list, can accommodate vegans, vegetarians, and omnivores.

---

180   This list is derived from USDA National Nutrient Database for Standard Reference, Release 18 http://www/ars.usda.gov/services/docs.htm?docid=9673

181   http://www.healthvitaminsguide.com/minerals/sulfur.htm

Table 4
Vitamin and Mineral Food Sources

Vegetables	Vitamin(s)	Mineral(s)	Beans (legumes)	Vitamin(s)	Mineral(s)
carrots	A		lentils	B_9	phosphorus, potassium, iron, molybdenum
cabbage, bok choi	K	calcium, sulfur			
sweet potato	A	potassium	lima beans	B_3, B_9	manganese, potassium, magnesium
winter squash	A	potassium	black (turtle) beans	B_1, B_9,	iron
avocado[6]	B_2, B_7		peanut	B_3, B_7, E	manganese, copper, zinc, phosphorus, magnesium
asparagus	B_2, E				
potato	B_5, C	chromium, calcium, iodine	peas (green)	A, B_1, B_5	molybdenum, nickel
yogurt	B_2, B_5, B_{12}	calcium, phosphorus	cashews[6]	B_7	zinc, copper, iron, molybdenum
egg	B_2, B_7	iodine, sulfur			
broccoli	B_9, C		chickpeas (garbanzos)	B_9	zinc, calcium
kale	A, K	calcium	white (navy) beans		calcium, potassium, zinc, iodine, manganese, molybdenum, nickel
onions	A, K	sulfur			
okra	A, B_9, K	calcium, manganese			
collard greens	A, B_1, B_9, K	calcium	kidney beans		iron

Table 4
Vitamin and Mineral Food Sources

mustard greens	A	calcium	soy beans, soy milk[7]	B_1,B_2, B_9, D, E	calcium, magnesium, phosphorus, iron,
dandelion greens	B_1,K	calcium	**Fruits**	**Vitamin(s)**	**Mineral(s)**
beet greens	K	calcium, magnesium, potassium	grapefruit	B_5	
turnip greens	B_9,	calcium	peaches	A	potassium
celery		chloride	orange (juice)	C, D	chromium
mushrooms	B_2, B_3, B_5, D	copper	apricots	A	potassium
spinach	A, E, K	magnesium, potassium, manganese	banana	B_6	potassium, chromium
Grains	**Vitamin(s)**	**Mineral(s)**	cantaloupe		potassium
brown rice	B_5, B_6	manganese,	**Nuts**	**Vitamin(s)**	**Mineral(s)**
barley	B_6	magnesium, phosphorus, copper, iron, manganese	almonds[6]	B_2, B_7	calcium, molybdenum
oat bran	B_1, B_5,	magnesium, iron, selenium	walnuts[7]		molybdenum
bulgur	B_3,B_5,	phosphorus, manganese	hazelnuts	B_7,E	
Dairy, Eggs	**Vitamin(s)**	**Mineral(s)**	sunflower seeds[6]	B_5,E	phosphorus[3]
cheese	B_7, B_{12}	calcium, phosphorus,	Brazil nuts[6]	B_1	selenium

Table 4
Vitamin and Mineral Food Sources

milk	B_1, B_5, B_{12}	calcium, phosphorus,	**Fish**	**Vitamin(s)**	**Mineral(s)**
Meat	**Vitamin(s)**	**Mineral(s)**	sardines	B_{12}	calcium, phosphorus, iodine
liver (beef, chicken)	A, B_2, B_7	copper	oysters	B_{12}	zinc
beef	B_3, B_{12}	phosphorus, zinc, copper, chromium, iron, selenium	halibut	B_3,	magnesium, phosphorus, selenium
chicken	B_3, B_5[4], B_6, B_{12}	phosphorus, zinc, iron[5], selenium	salmon	B_{12},D	calcium, selenium

Notes:
1 Soy milk or soy yogurt would have Vitamin D only if it were "fortified" with Vitamin D.
2 It is only the broccoli leaves, not the florets, that provide Vitamin A.
3 Sunflower seeds has phosphorus and phytic acid. The phytic acid prevents about 50% or less of the attachment of phosphorus by the human digestive system. The bacteria lactobacillus acidophilus and lactobacillus casei, resident in the human mouth, neutralize that part of the phytic acid. If the colony were reinforced by the eating of yogurt, either milk or soy, more of the phytic acid would be neutralized, and more of the phosphorus would be gained by the human body.
4 The white meat of the chicken provides Vitamin B_5.
5 The dark meat of the chicken provides iron.
6 Avocados, almonds, Brazil nuts, cashews, and sunflower seeds also have linoleic acid (omega 6) and no α-linolenic acid (omega 3).
7 Soy beans and walnuts have both linoleic acid (omega 6) and α-linolenic acid (omega 3).

Table 1 on pages 14 and 15 provides the fatty acid content percentages for some of the foods listed in the table above. Table 5, just below, restates the information for dietary minerals provided in pages 65 to 76 above. But Table 5 distributes the foods associated with each dietary mineral and vitamin according to whether it is a vegetable or fruit, a grain or nut, a bean, dairy or egg, or meat or fish. This provides alternatives for people who may want to plan their meals by this table. It also indicates for vegans and vegetarians, which foods qualify under their strictures. As was said with respect to Table 4, as Vitamin B_{12} can only be gained through the eating of animal meat or animal products, vegans should seek to get their required Vitamin B_{12} through supplements.

Again, it should be made explicit that only the major sources of each vitamin or mineral is listed.

Table 5
Vitamins and Minerals and the Foods Containing Each

Vitamin or Mineral	Vegetables & Fruits	Grains & Nuts	Beans (Legumes)	Dairy & Eggs	Meat & Fish
A **Retinol**	carrots, onions sweet potato winter squash kale, collard greens, spinach, okra, mustard greens, apricots peaches		peas (green)		liver cod liver oil
B₁ **Thiamin**	Spinach orange cantaloupe yeast	brown rice whole wheat bread wheat germ Brazil nuts pecans	lentils peas	milk egg	pork
B2 **Riboflavin**	avocado, mushrooms, asparagus.		soy	yogurt egg	beef liver chicken liver

Table 5
Vitamins and Minerals and the Foods Containing Each

Vitamin or Mineral	Vegetables & Fruits	Grains & Nuts	Beans (Legumes)	Dairy & Eggs	Meat & Fish
B3 Niacin	mushrooms	bulgur	lima beans, peanut		beef, chicken, halibut
B5 Pantothenic Acid	potato, mushrooms grapefruit	brown rice, oat bran, bulgur	peas	yogurt milk	chicken
B6 Pyridoxal phosphate	banana	sunflow-er seeds			chicken salmon
B7 Biotin	avocado	almond hazelnut	cashews peanuts	egg cheese	liver
B9 Folic acid	okra, collard greens, broccoli, lturnip greens,		lentils, chickpeas (garbanzos) lima beans, black (turtle) beans, lima beans		
B12 Cobalamin				yogurt, milk' cheese	sardines, salmon oysters beef chicken
C Ascorbic acid	orange, broccoli, potato				
D Cholecalcif-erol1	orange juice[2], mushrooms	cereal[2]	soy milk[2]	cow's milk[2]	salmon

Table 5
Vitamins and Minerals and the Foods Containing Each

Vitamin or Mineral	Vegetables & Fruits	Grains & Nuts	Beans (Legumes)	Dairy & Eggs	Meat & Fish
E Alpha-Tocopherol	asparagus, spinach	hazelnut sunflow-er seeds	peanuts, soy beans		
K Phylloqui-none	kale, cabbage, spinach, onions, okra, beet greens, dandelion greens				
Calcium	turnip greens, bok choy, potato, collard greens, kale, okra, mustard greens, dandelion greens, beet greens	almonds	chick peas (garbanzos), navy (white) beans, soy beans	milk yogurt cheese	salmon, sardines
Chloride[3]	celery, tomatoes	rye			
Magnesium	spinach, okra, beet greens	oat bran, barley	soy beans, lima beans		halibut
Phosphorus		barley, bulgur, sunflower seeds	lentils[4] peanuts[4] soy beans	milk, yogurt, cheese	beef, chicken, halibut, sardines

Table 5
Vitamins and Minerals and the Foods Containing Each

Vitamin or Mineral	Vegetables & Fruits	Grains & Nuts	Beans (Legumes)	Dairy & Eggs	Meat & Fish
Potassium	sweet potato beet greens winter squash		lentils lima beans		
Sodium					
Zinc			cashews, peanuts, chickpeas (garbanzos), navy (white) beans		oysters, beef, chicken
Chromium	potato				beef
Cobalt					
Copper	mushrooms	barley	cashews, peanuts		liver
Iodine	potato seaweed		navy (white) beans	egg	sardines
Iron		barley, oat bran	cashews, kidney beans, black (turtle) beans, lentils, soy beans		beef chicken
Manganese	spinach, okra	brown rice, barley, bulgur	lima beans, white (navy) beans, peanuts		
Molyb-denum			lentils, peas, cashews, navy (white) beans		
Nickel			peas, navy (white) beans		

Table 5
Vitamins and Minerals and the Foods Containing Each

Vitamin or Mineral	Vegetables & Fruits	Grains & Nuts	Beans (Legumes)	Dairy & Eggs	Meat & Fish
Selenium		Brazil nuts, oat bran		milk	salmon halibut chicken beef
Sulfur	cabbage, onions			egg	

NOTES: 1. Cholecalciferol is made in the bare human skin, without sun block, when it is struck with the ultraviolet light of the sun. However, people in northern latitudes, or anywhere if they don't get out to the sun sufficiently, will have to augment their supply of Vitamin D with supplements or animal foods, mainly fish, which contain it.
2. Orange juice, cereal, soy milk, and cow's milk only has Vitamin D3, cholecalciferol, if it has been added as a 'reinforcing' supplement. This will be indicated on the package, which will say that Vitamin D has been added.
3. Chloride can be readily attained through table or sea salt. The normal salting of food, not heavy, is more than sufficient for the intake of chloride.
4. Almonds and whole wheat bread have phosphorus and phytic acid. The phytic acid prevents about 50% or less of the attachment of phosphorus by the human digestive system. The bacteria lactobacillus acidophilus and lactobacillus casei, resident in the human mouth, neutralize that part of the phytic acid. If the colony were reinforced by the eating of yogurt, either milk or soy, more of the phytic acid would be neutralized, and more of the phosphorus would be gained by the human body.

Aside from the different eating styles, one must still be aware of which foods are healthy. In the American food production system, it is quite possible, actually very easy, to select a vegan diet that is unhealthy. Vegetables grown with manure secured from factory farms will have hormones and may be imbalanced in minerals. They also may have harmful pathogens. If the manure came from cattle feed lots, the vegetables are likely to have a very high dose of phosphorus. Cattle, evolved as grass eating Bovidae, have no way to overcome the phytic acid in corn. Therefore, the phosphorus content of corn passes right through. That which doesn't go down the stream, into the Mississippi River, and out to the Gulf, where the waters are eutrofied, will be in the manure sold to vegetable farmers. Farmers who buy feedlot manure probably also douse their monocrops with insecticides. These poisoned vegetables are sold through your local supermarket, a place you will not want to buy unpackaged food, unless it is identified as 'organic' in a separate section. But such sections are often not broadly stocked.

Healthy vegetables, which we should all eat, are, fortunately, locally available to most people in the country. Near most cities, near most towns, are small, local farmers, many of whom grow organically. They sell their vegetables in the summer either from the farm, or through a local farmers' market, or through a food cooperative. If you buy your produce directly from the farm, you know what you are getting. Purchasing from a local farmers' market is not that simple. The local organic farmer or farmers will be there, but one or more commercial farmers may be there as well. Just because they are selling their feedlot fertilized, insecticided produce at a farmers' market does not make that food healthy. So, it behooves you to know who the venders at your local farmers' market are.

Many cities and towns have a food coop. These are generally committed to healthy food. They may not all understand all of the, or even the major, threats to health there are, but even if they focus on food that is certified organic, and produce that is grown without insecticide, that is a pretty good indicator of local, healthy food. Many food coops do not have a produce section. Thus you will have to return to the farmers' market, or patronize a Whole Foods supermarket. This is the one supermarket chain which has a commitment to healthier food. But one must still be aware. Some Whole Foods stores sell both 'commercial' and 'organic' food. For reasons already gone over, you should stay away from commercial food. The organic food, particularly produce, will probably be from a fairly local farm or farms in the summer. But they also import organic foods from California to the East and Midwest, as well as from Mexico, Guatemala, and Chile. If the food is 'organic,' though from Mexico, it is still your best indicator of healthy produce.

If you buy packaged food, you should read the ingredients. Beware of salt, especially too much, of preservatives, of taste enhancers, such as monosodium glutamate (MSG). If the ingredient list lists a number of items you can't recognize, or chemicals with long names, remember your intention is to buy food. If there are things you cannot recognize, and long chemical names, it is best to avoid it. It may not be food, despite what it says on the package. Of course the certified organic label is the safest. But if it is not available, or you want something else, the best thing is to carefully read the ingredients.

If you do want to eat meat, you should look for grass fed beef, free range chickens and turkeys, and pasture raised goats or pigs. You may know a farm which raises and sells grass fed beef near you. If you are not aware of such a farm, there, nevertheless, probably are one or several such farms reasonably close to you. To find such farms consult http://eatwild.com. This lists the grass fed beef, free range poultry, and pastured goat farms in your state; so, you can find one or more near where you live. If you don't live anywhere near any listing in eatwild.com, and you live in the continental 48 states of the USA, Puerto Rico, or Canada, you can order grass fed beef, poultry, pork, goats, lambs, bison, or rabbits from http://slankersgrassfedmeats.com/index.htm.

So, eating healthfully involves eating plenty of green, leafy vegetables and other vegetables, all of which have not been raised with insecticide, or fertilized with feed lot manure. For beef, pork, chicken, turkey, or goats, get them from farms which raise the cattle on grass and hay, the pigs in outdoor pens where they get to root in the ground, chickens and turkeys on a range, where they get to scratch and eat insects, and goats on a pasture where they can munch on grass and shrubbery. And for package goods, read the ingredients very carefully.

8 – The Proper Health Practitioner

THE MOST IMPORTANT SKILL of the health practitioner is diagnoses. When a person comes to a health practitioner with the claim of feeling ill, who seems to be malfunctioning, or in a state of physiological degeneration, it is incumbent upon the health practitioner to determine the nature and cause of the condition. This is not simple. There are about 100 billion cells, about one trillion commensal bacteria, a great number of potentially pathogenic bacteria on the skin, numerous enzymes, organs, and processes. Given this complexity, with very few exceptions, there is ambiguity in the exhibition of an illness. After all, there are far fewer ways a person can exhibit illness.

But the incumbency persists. A diagnoses must be made. Treatment cannot be decided until such a diagnoses is made. And it is no adverse reflection on the skill of a health practitioner if she, from time to time, makes a misdiagnoses. This may become apparent upon the lack of response to the treatment, a re-interpretation of a patient's response in her history, or the emergence of some other data. A change in the treatment is then prescribed. But, if an ameliorative response is to be given, a diagnoses must be made.

Of course, for serious illnesses, for obscure presentations, there is the examination of blood and urine samples. Such analysis may reveal an absence or severe shortage of selenium, or pyridoxamine, or, pertinent to the current reality, a severe shortage of eicosapentaenoic acid (EPA) and docosahexaenoic acid (DHA). The deficiency of selenium may indicate other deficiencies, and further analysis would have to be made. But to deal with the selenium deficiency, the health practitioner would prescribe Brazil nuts, enriched noodles, and whole wheat bread. If they eat fish, then free swimming halibut would be prescribed. For the deficiency of pyridoxamine, Vitamin B$_6$ tablets would be prescribed, along with the advice to include bananas and baked potatoes in their diet. For the deficiencies of EPA and DHA, several tablespoons daily of fresh, unrefined, and unfiltered flax oil would be prescribed.

As may be surmised from the preceding paragraph, it is the contention of this book that the most common cause of illness is a deficiency in an essential vitamin, fat, or mineral, or a combination thereof. The only other causes of illness are the ingestion or absorption of a toxin, or the attack of a pathogen, particularly one for which there is no immune response. A small minority of persons also have a strong genetic determinant of particular diseases. In this essay, these cases are ignored. It has rather been the attempt in the earlier chapters to demonstrate that most of the disease in this disease ridden country can be attributed to deficiency, particularly a deficiency of omega 3 fatty acids. This refers to hypertension, ischemic heart disease, neoplastic tumors, rheumatoid arthritis, other autoimmune conditions, and depression. There may be others. But this accounts for a good deal of the disease in this country, and all of it can be attributed to the over consumption of corn.

Evolution produces healthy specimens. They are the ones most capable of survival and reproduction. The normal state of a human being is to be healthy and alert, as is that of a fox, a golden eagle, and a sperm whale. And that human being, eating the diet she was evolved to eat, omnivoric or vegetarian, will remain healthy. Even without biochemical and dietitian training, she could assume that all of the food elements she needs for healthful living are in her diet, and for the most part of human history, until the last 50 odd years, that was true. And the elimination of the factory farms could return this to a healthy nation, and reduce national health costs by as much as 80%.

There are, unfortunately, major, moneyed powers that would spend money to maintain the current situation. Perhaps the most powerful, the most moneyed of these is the pharmaceutical industry. They are getting richer daily with this system. It doesn't seem to matter to them that the system is causing 80 million people to be diseased, and causing 400,000 deaths by disease annually. The most important thing to them is that they are making a lot of money.

So, let's discuss the pharmaceutical industry. They are very major players in the current system, and they are part of the problem. If we succeed in eliminating the factory farms, it will only occur by first defeating and reducing the pharmaceutical firms. They make a lot of money with factory farms. They deliver tons of antibiotics to factory farms, and that is money. You might object and mention the fact that the reckless distribution of antibiotics is causing strain after strain of antibiotic resistant bacteria, and that, after a while, the antibiotics will be ineffective. But the pharmaceutical response is that the "after a while" will take care of itself, that in the meantime they are making money. That the name of the game is making money, and they are winning at that game; they are making lots of money.

Now many of the readers of this book, and others, will say that they are not involved in any game. That what they want is a safe, healthy, and happy life. But they are not the heads of the pharmaceutical firms, are they?

The pharmaceutical industry can be traced back about 120 years ago to the patent medicine vendors of the cities and towns of this country then. They hawked their patent medicines as remedies of common maladies, of coughs, upset stomach, lethargy. Americans at that time were a healthy people. There were not many serious illnesses. But there were respiratory problems, especially for those working in dusty conditions and in mines. There were also afflictions of the back, and other pains and conditions. Those are what the patent medicines were claimed to help.

It was not easy for the patent medicine vendors. They had strong competition. There were people vending herbal remedies, seed oils, and ointments. These vendors had a lot of responsiveness among the people. For thousands of years people have used herbal remedies for their various ills. They learned, over thousands of years, which plants, which leaves, which berries were helpful for which illness or injury. This was the basis of medicine for thousands of years, all over the world, in North and South America, in Africa, in Europe, and in Asia, and the vendors of these natural remedies naturally received a sympathetic ear.

But the patent medicine vendors had a new, modern line of remedies, and they were determined, even desperate, to get them accepted. They had no historically established, time tested medicines; nevertheless they argued that these were, in fact, new, scientific, especially formulated medicines. Given the competition, they also had a second line of argument, that the herbal remedies, the ointments, were ineffective, that these natural remedy guys were just trying to fool you; they had nothing which would help you. After a while, it became apparent to the patent medicine vendors that the negative argument was more effective.

The negative argument got a powerful boost when they attacked natural remedy of vendors who were hawking an ointment from California. This ointment came from China, and was used by the Chinese laborers who worked on the transcontinental railway. This was grunt work, and many workers got bursitis and arthritis, and applied this ointment for relief. It was so effective, that the natural remedy vendors took it and were offering it all over the country. It was called Snake Oil Liniment,[182] and the patent medicine vendors latched on to that. Although snake oil was also used in Egyptian medicine, the European derived population of this country had never heard of such substance being used as medicine. It sounded strange, and unnatural. That is all the patent medicine hawkers needed. They ridiculed the snake oil and snake oil salesmen as phony and fraudulent. They contrasted that unquestionably fake snake oil with their patented medicine, patented by the government.

And it worked. To this day, snake oil connotes fraud and fakery. Even President George W. Bush, used the term "snake oil salesmen" to castigate those who were arguing for renewable energy, and who were opposed to his proposal to drill for oil off shore the Eastern states.

The patent medicine vendors evolved into pharmaceutical firms. Patent medicine cum pharmaceutical industry got a boost with the passage of the Federal Food, Drug, and Cosmetic Act of 1938, which required the administration of certain, tested drugs only by prescription by a licensed physician. After the Second World War, with sulfa drugs having been developed, and used, and other variations and formulations to be developed, the pharmaceutical industry took off. The factory farm system was starting, and the newly developed antibiotic drugs were called for. The pharmaceutical firms poured the antibiotics into the factory farms, and made much money. These were the same antibiotics they sold in ointments or to the public and human physicians. Lots of money. And they used their money intelligently. They inserted pharmaceutical components into the curricula of medical schools, to guarantee that the "physicians" authorized to prescribe medications would be schooled in their pharmaceutical philosophy. They launched lobbyists, and bought congressmen. They bought magazine and television advertisements for their drugs, even for prescription drugs. Thus, they could pressure physicians. And, with a sympathetic president and administration, they could even control the FDA. Success is definitely sweet. And you know why? Because they could make lots of money.

---

182   Cf. http://en.wikipedia.org/wiki/Snake_oil

There is also the revealing fact that during the rise of the pharmaceutical medical culture during the last 50 years, this country has become the most diseased country of all of the countries with medical records in the world. Fully one fourth of the adults in this country have a serious disease, and annually 400,000 prematurely die of ischemic heart disease. Doesn't this reflect badly on the pharmaceutical medical culture? Are the pharmaceutical firms concerned? Does the reader think they are concerned about the health of the American people? You misunderstand these folks. They are concerned about one thing; making money. Diseased people? They can sell many more pharmaceuticals. They can make lots of money.

There still are, have always been, natural health practitioners. Nowadays, these practitioners are trained in biochemistry and dietetics, and practice an orthomolecular form of healthcare. And how do the *nouveau* patent medicine hawkers, the pharmaceutical firms regard these natural health practitioners? Well, they are all snake oil salesmen.

In 1989, a nutrition-oriented medical doctor from California decided to find out what snake oil contains. He obtained a sample of the oil from San Francisco's Chinatown, had it analyzed, and found that it contains 75% unidentified carrier material, presumably for emulsifying the snake oil and helping to transport it through the skin. It also contains camphor. The remaining 25% of the product is oil from Chinese water snakes, which contains 20% of the important omega 3 derivative eicosapentaenoic acid (EPA) as well as 48% myristic acid (14:0), 10% stearic acid (18:0), 14% oleic acid (18:1w9), and 7% linoleic (18:2w6) plus arachidonic (20:4w6) acids. At 20% EPA, Chinese water snake is the richest known natural source of the parent of series 3 prostaglandins, which inhibit the production of pro-inflammatory series 2 prostaglandins. Like essential fatty acids and their other derivatives, EPA can be absorbed through our skin. Salmon oil, the next-best source of EPA, contains a maximum of only 18% EPA. Other fish oils contain less.[183]

Chinese snake oil liniment is still sold throughout the country in Chinese shops and Chinese pharmacies. It still works, as it always has, to relieve joint pain. So, if you suffer from bursitis, rub the snake oil on the

---

183   Erasmus, Udo. *Fats that Heal; Fats that Kill*, 17th edition, 2006, pp 268-269.

shoulder area, and do so daily for five consecutive days. During this period do not lift the arm, and keep if from lifting anything heavy. After a week, the bursitis should be healed.

The physician referenced above is Dr. Richard Kunin. He

> submitted a report of his findings on the ingredients of snake oil to the *New England Journal of Medicine*. They were unwilling to publish it. Might it be more important to keep the image from being tarnished than to disseminate accurate information? If they were wrong about snake oil, what else should we question about the patent medicines-cum-drugs approach?[184]

Now how does a proper health care, an orthomolecular health care, practitioner diagnose and treat one or more cases of deficiency disease? Again, the assumption is that a body not afflicted with a toxin or under attack by a pathogen, would be perfectly healthy, unless there were a deficiency in one or more of the 13 vitamins, and/or one or more of the 16 dietary minerals, or one or both of the essential fatty acids. Of course a small minority of people may exhibit some dysfunction due to the inheritance of a genetic mutation. There is a large number of such conditions. Some are fatal in early youth; others, with compensatory adjustment, can function normally, or very nearly so. These people do require medical attention, but the number of genetically induced diseases is around one per cent. I wish to restrict our discussion to acquired conditions or illnesses.

So, a proper health care practitioner would diagnose a patient brought to her, to determine the precise deficiency or deficiencies. The object of this diagnoses and health care is to cure the disease; to restore the person, if possible, to full health. If the patient shows conditions indicative of a deficiency in alpha-linolenic acid (omega 3), and analysis confirms this, the treatment will include such fatty acid, probably initially in large doses. But analysis may also indicate an over consumption of sodium, a deficiency in magnesium, and a deficiency in certain vitamins. The full treatment would have to encompass all of those substances, and the practitioner may also suggest some changes in the patient's diet. This may also involve a concomitant change in the patient's life style, but if recovery is the goal, then all of that would be required.

This differs fundamentally from the pharmaceutical medical approach. I say "pharmaceutical medical," but the intent here is to concentrate on

---

184   *Ibid.*, p. 269.

the drugs which have been used for the several deficiency conditions, or diseases, as the patent medicine hawkers cum pharmaceutical firms call them. Before proceeding, let me state that the philosophy of the pharmaceutical industry seems to be that diseases simply occur, and it is the appropriate response to ameliorate the unfortunate person, and to try to prolong that person's life. Let's now look at cholesterol. There is the condition of hypercholesterolemia, which refers to the presence of abnormally high levels of cholesterol in the bloodstream, particularly high levels of low density lipoprotein (LDL). The University of Maryland Medical Center identifies hypercholesterolemia as having a measured blood cholesterol of 240 mg/dl or higher.[185] This is also referred to as the "high risk" level, because it is correlated with the incidence of heart attack in many people. And aside from, and preliminary to, heart attacks is cardiovascular disease (CVD), and particularly coronary artery disease (CAD), the initial presentation of which, for up to one-third of patients is sudden death.[186] This makes physicians particularly anxious to control CVD/CAD, and hypercholesterolemia seems to be a handle for such control.

But it is an error to focus on hypercholesterolemia. It is exceedingly unlikely that a person would present hypercholesterolemia, and not have other evidence of neglect and abuse. Typically, a patient measuring 253 mg/dl is also overweight, deficient in alpha-linolenic acid (omega 3), Vitamin B$_3$ (Niacin, Nicotinic acid), Vitamin C, and probably other vitamins, as well as certain essential minerals, and has very probably consumed a quantity of soft toxins. I refer to transfats as "soft toxins" because the body cannot use them for any construction, immunological, or other operational purpose. It can only burn them for energy, and any excess is simply put in LDLs. Hypercholesterolemia would be a symptom of these deficiencies. But unless the deficiencies are addressed, simply bringing down the cholesterol level, a large portion of which is probably low density lipoprotein (LDL), will not save the client from CVD and a heart attack. But there are physicians, heavily influenced by pharmaceutical firms, who believe that the LDL cholesterol level has to be urgently brought down, and who are aware that there is a drug that can do that. Of course there is a drug, and that drug

---

185   http://www.umm.edu/altmed/articles/hypercholesterolemia-000084.htm

186   Bunzell, J.D.; Davidson, M.; Furberg, C.D.; Goldberg, R.B.; Howard, B.V.; Stein, J. G.; and Witztum, J.L. "Lipoprotein Management in Patients With Cardiometabolic Risk," Journal of the American College of Cardiology, 51:1512-1524 (27 March 2008), p. 1513.

is a statin, more specifically, it is probably atorvastatin, which is marketed in this country as Lipitor. There are other statins, simvastatin, marketed as Zocor; lovastatin, marketed as Mevacor; and pravastatin, marketed as Pravachol, but with 2006 sales of $12.9 billion, Lipitor is the largest selling drug in the world[187], and, therefore, is probably the one prescribed in the hypothetical case being discussed.

What a statin, such as atorvastatin, does is to interfere with an enzyme in the HMG-CoA reductase pathway, which is the process in which each cell produces cholesterol. In a normally sized person, about one gram of high density lipoprotein (HDL) cholesterol is synthesized each day. The body normally synthesizes high density lipoproteins to be used in repairing and maintaining cell membranes, and to form scabs where surface injury occurs. This synthesis occurs in many cells, with 20 -25% of it occurring in the liver. HMG-CoA reductase is the enzyme, which converts 3-hydroxy-3-methylglutaryl-CoA (HMG-CoA) into mevalonic acid, which is at the head of a nine step process to form cholesterol. A statin drug, any of them, acts against HMG-CoA reductase to prevent it from forming mevalonic acid. Very large doses (80 mg/day) of atorvastatin will reduce 51% of the mevalonic acid from forming. Since mevalonic acid is at the head of a nine step process to form cholesterol, 51% of the cholesterol will not be formed.

But it is not that simple. Mevalonic acid is also at the head of a six step process to form ubiquinon and dolichol. Ubiquinone (Coenzyme Q_{10}) is an oil-soluble vitamin-like substance present in the mitochondria. It is a component of the electron transport chain and participates in aerobic cellular respiration, generating energy in the form of ATP. Ninety-five percent of the human body's energy is generated this way.[188] Therefore it is present in high numbers in all tissues and organs which use energy frequently, the heart, the liver, muscles, and the neuronic system, including the brain.

Dolichol refers to any of a group of long-chain mostly unsaturated organic compounds which are made up of varying numbers of similarly structured carbon-hydrogen units terminating in a unit which contains an alcohol functional group.[189] It works in each cell with proteins manufactured in response to DNA directives, and directs them to their

---

187   http://en.wikipedia.org/wiki/Atorvastatin

188   http://en.wikipedia.org/wiki/Coenzyme_Q10

189   http://en.wikipedia.org/wiki/Dolichol

proper target, ensuring that the cells respond correctly to genetically programmed instruction.

Thus, statin, at 80 mg/day, also reduces ubiquinone and dolichol to 78% of their normal production. This has ramifications for the maintenance and operation of the entire body. Even with a prescription for 40 mg/day, the effect is to reduce cholesterol, ubiquinon, and dolichol to 49% of the normal production. This has implications, after months of use, for muscular and neurologic dysfunction.

It should be recalled that, along with the reduction in ubiquinone and dolichol, a statin interferes with and reduces a cell's own produced HDL cholesterol, which is produced for the maintenance of cell membranes, and for use in forming scabs to seal an open wound. This process has nothing to do with the level of LDL or VLDL in the circulatory system, which came there by way of diet. The danger a person has of thrombosis and heart attack does not derive from its normal cellular HMG-CoA reductase pathway procedure. The danger comes from the eating of substances which produce LDLs and VLDLs in the blood stream, which are not 'burned off' by exercise. There is no pharmaceutical drug which addresses and reduces those.

So the cholesterol which forms hypercholesterolemia is not HDL cholesterol. It is generally low density, or very low density lipoproteins (LDL or VLDL) cholesterol. The rational way to design a therapy for our hypercholesterolemic patient, with a severely high cholesterol reading, is, first, to prohibit the consumption of transfats, in margarine and vegetable shortening which contains transfats, and high temperature fried, especially deep fried, foods, which produce transfats. Hypercholesterolemia, as caused by a large amount of LDLs, has been demonstrated to result from the consumption of partially hydrogenated vegetable oils, which form transfats.[190] In addition, alpha-linolenic acid, high doses of Vitamin C (2,000 mg/day), N-acetyl cysteine (a mucus dissolving agent, which acts as a prophylaxis for obstructive pulmonary disease), niacin (Vitamin B_3), carnitine (an ammonium compound required for the transport of fatty acids into mitochondria) , lysine (an essential amino acid with a role in catalysis), proline (an amino acid which is synthesized by humans, with a role in catalysis), magnesium, co-enzyme Q_{10} (ubiquinone), and others would be

---

190   Erasmus, Udo. Fats that Heal; Fats that Kill, 17th printing, 2006, p. 111 also The Mayo Clinic, in its report "Trans fat: Avoid this Cholesterol Double Whammy, which may be found at http://www.mayoclinic.com/print/trans-fat/CL00032/METHOD=print .

prescribed and administered. If the consumption of trans fats is terminated immediately, the prescribed nutrients taken, and healthy dietary guidelines are followed, the LDL level, as measured by the cholesterol test, will immediately decline. There is no need for a statin, or any such interference in the bodily processes. What is needed is to get the body to function normally, and for this, it needs a full set of the essential fats, vitamins, and minerals. If a person has degenerated to the point where they can be identified as suffering from hypercholesterolemia, then some abnormally large dose of core nutrients have to be administered. If the cholesterol level was very high, and the patient's cholesterol does not seem to move, even as treatment begins, then meat, and other animal products, including eggs, milk, and butter, will have to be eliminated from the diet. As all external cholesterol comes from animal products, this will guarantee reduction in cholesterol. Once the cholesterol level is normal, the nutrient doses can cease. But continued health requires that the patient cease the ingestion of toxins and of an inadequate diet. Of course that is a description of the current normal American diet, but that normal American diet has caused deficiency disease in every other adult in the country. So the patient, if she desires to be healthy, will have to take the extra effort to seek out healthy foods, including greens, not contaminated with insecticide, and healthy oils with both essential fatty acids. It is a testimony of the perverse state the current food production system is in North America, that extra effort has to be expended to find healthy food.

Of course, the prescription nutrition listed in the previous paragraph to address the hypothetical patient are only illustrative. A particular prescription for a particular person would have to be pursuant from that person's diagnosis.

But some physicians confuse the administration of a drug with therapy, and they keep a person on a statin for years, in some cases, over ten years. For a number of these physicians, no dietary prescriptions are made. The "therapy" is the taking of a statin drug. But the question has to be asked: How does a statin drug cure the patient? The obvious answer is that it does nothing to cure the patient. It controls the wrong cholesterol level, and at a cost, over a number of years, of the physical and mental degeneration of the patient. We will look at a couple of other drugs to demonstrate this pattern, but patent medicine hawkers cum pharmaceutical firms have never been in the business of curing patients. They are in the business of selling drugs. And, in the case of Pfizer with Lipitor (atorvastatin), it is bringing in $13 billion a year.

Have physicians who prescribe the continuous taking of a statin for years forgotten that part of the Hippocratic Oath which says they should "do no harm?" For those who put themselves in and remain in the thrall of pharmaceutical firms, they will not be able to avoid doing harm. They should reflect mightily on that.

We have discussed hypercholesterolemia. Now let us discuss breast cancer, after which we will discuss depression.

Breast cancer is a very high incidence disease in the United States. It affects both men and women, but it is overwhelmingly a women's affliction. Breast cancer among women in North America has the highest incidence rates in the world, and is the second most common cause of cancer death. Women in the United States have a 12.5% lifetime chance of developing invasive breast cancer, and a 3% chance of dying from it.

A number of medical researchers and physicians contend that cancer, including breast cancer, and sometimes explicitly breast cancer, is determined by genes. This does not seem to be an adequate explanation. North America has the highest rate of incidence of any region in the world. Except for a small minority of Native Americans, the genetic composition of the other Americans all hail from Europe, Africa, and Asia. And Europe, Africa, and Asia all have lower rates of incidence. Western Europe, which shares some of the types of food of North America, has a rate which is 87% of the North American rate. The rate for Northern Europe is 81%, Southern Europe is 62%, and Eastern Europe is 54% of the North American rate. Sub-Saharan Africa has a rate of 24%, and East Asia has a rate 20% of the North American rate. So what do these medical researchers and physicians contend? That the determinant genes work intermittently in Asia or Africa, or that they work sporadically in Europe? Such a position would be difficult to sustain, I would think.

The determination to find the genetic source of disease is derivative of pharmaceutical thinking. The operating assumption is that disease is 'normal,' that it is the unfortunate lot of humanity to suffer disease and frequent early death. Thus, it is a mercy that pharmaceutical firms can develop drugs to relieve the misery. This manner of thinking is an offense to truth, reason, and reality.

Given that there are about 26,000 genes in the human genome, it is a near certainty that one can find a gene or combination of genes that relate to any physiological or behavior outcome. But it is not at all reasonable to research the genome as the definitive treatment of a disease. The overwhelming majority of 'diseases' are expressions of degeneration, of deficiency in one or more factors of life, or a surfeit of the same. The conditions referred to as diseases by the large majority of afflicted can be 'cured' by the application of a orthomolecular, dietary treatment. This has been described above, and will be described again below. So, it is medically critical to look elsewhere before looking at the genome with the object of curing most 'diseases.'

This is not to say that some people do not have predispositional genes for cancer or some other condition. I would contend that people worldwide have a number of such predispositional genes. And, in fairness, cancer is a very ancient disease; definitive evidence of its incidence has been found in Egyptian mummies, and other ancient archeological sites. There is incidence of breast cancer in areas where we must assume that there are not significant dietary deficiencies. So, there seems to be a genetic basis for a certain incidence of breast cancer. If we look at Table 3 on page 23, we see that eastern Asia has an incidence of breast cancer of .018% of the population. South central Asia and Sub-Saharan Africa have rates, each, of .022%. Thus, for practical reasons we may assume that genes account for around .02% of breast cancer cases worldwide. That still leaves North America with .09%, Western Europe with .078%, Northern Europe with .073%, Southern Europe with .056%, and Eastern Europe with .05%. In these areas, a majority of cases has to be attributable to a factor or factors other than genes. The contention here is that diet is the determinative factor. Because of the deficient and toxic ridden food supply in North America, many people, after unwittingly abusing their bodies for years, suffer systemic degeneration, of which breast cancer is one symptom. You don't find much cancer among newborns, or young children. It is rare among teenagers and people in their twenties. The incidence of breast cancer increases as the person gets older. By the late thirties, by the forties and fifties it is almost epidemic in incidence. This suggest the factor of dietary deficiency. It had to wait until the body degenerated to the point where the immune system was severely disabled, the liver was only partially functioning, and the operational capacity of the cells of the other vital organs is severely reduced. In such a condition of degeneration, if there are microbes which play a role in neoplastic cancer, they would be able to freely take their place; they wouldn't even be challenged by the compromised immune system.

In terms of orthomolecular therapy, unless the person's system has degenerated to the point of imminent collapse, metastasis being one indicator of that, the appropriate response to breast cancer is to provide the patient with the essential nutrients she has neglected, usually with initially substantial doses, and then direct the patient to henceforth eat healthy food, which would include all of the essential fats, vitamins, and minerals. Specifically, she would be prescribed fresh, unrefined flax oil (five tablespoons daily, initially, then three, then a maintenance dose of two tablespoons, daily), Vitamins C, B_3, potassium, and iodine, in large initial doses. She would also be counseled to eat fresh vegetables, including greens, whole grains, and a decreased consumption of animal products. "Digestive enzymes are commonly used in natural and orthomolecular treatments of cancer."[191] And if microbes are found to be participants in tumor growth, once the immune system is re-invigorated, it will take out such microbes, and not permit any others to operate in the system. Or, in the case of pleomorphic microbes, which assume a virulent form in the presence of a severe imbalance of fatty acids, these will again assume a benign form in a person with a regenerated, reconstituted body who consumes a healthy proportion of essential fatty acids.

Of course, if she is the one of the two in a thousand whose breast cancer is the product of malfunctioning or mutated genes, this orthomolecular treatment will not suffice. But for 76% of the cases in North America, the orthomolecular treatment is indicated.

The research sustaining this prescription has already been cited on page 15 above. The operant summary statement is:

> Diets rich in omega-6 polyunsaturated fatty acids stimulate the growth and metasteses of transplantable mammary carcinomas in rodents, whereas fish oil-containing diets, rich in omega-3 fatty acids, suppress the growth of these mammary tumor cells.[192]

Within a few months of the treatment referenced above, the tumors will be eliminated; the cancer will be gone. After the treatment is finished, and the cancer is gone, and the patient continues to consume a healthy diet, her survival will no more be jeopardized. " Successful reversals of cancers, in which cancer totally disappeared and the person was still alive

---

191   Erasmus, Udo. Fats that Heal; Fats that Kill, 17th printing (2006), p.367.

192   Rose, D.P. and Connolly, J.M. "Effects of dietary omega-3 fatty acids on human breast cancer growth and metastases in nude mice," Journal of the National Cancer Institute, 1993 Nov 3;85(21):1743-7, found in http://www.ncbi.nlm.nih.gov/pubmed/8411258

an cancer-free 10, 20, 30, and even 40 years after the diagnosis of 'terminal' cancer was made, have been documented."[193]

Before we compare the orthomolecular method of healthcare with the pharmaceutical method, let us reiterate the premises of the orthomolecular, natural healthcare. Unless there is extreme maternal deprivation, a child starts life in a healthy state, receiving all of the nutrients she needs from her mother's milk. Then, if the child is reasonably active, and eats a healthy diet, which consists of both essential fatty acids, the 13 vitamins, and the 16 dietary minerals, and does not ingest toxins, she will continue to be healthy. If she maintains this diet as she gets older, and she continues to be reasonably active, she will be healthy throughout her life. So, the premises are that a person is normally healthy, and can be kept healthy with the breathing of adequate oxygen, exposure to adequate light, the drinking of adequate clean water, and the eating of wholesome food, comprehensive of both essential fatty acids, the 13 vitamins, and the 16 dietary minerals. If a person is chronically deficient in lysine, calcium absorption will decline, and she will eventually be diagnosed with osteoporosis. If a person is chronically deficient in alpha-linolenic acid she will suffer frequent inflammation and blood platelet aggregation. If she is also over abundant with linoleic acid, she will eventually be diagnosed with cancer, or rheumatoid arthritis, or some other autoimmune disease. And so forth. But it can be seen that the condition, because of the neglect of essential nutrients, is that of physiological degeneration. The so-called diseases, osteoporosis, rheumatoid arthritis, cancer, cardio vascular disease, hypercholesterolemia are all but symptoms of the state of degeneration. If the degeneration could be repaired by the restoration of the neglected essential nutrients, and the patient henceforth eats a wholesome, nutritionally comprehensive food, all of these diagnosed diseases will disappear.

Let's continue the example of a child born in 1942. In 1947, at five years of age, the child continues to receive healthful nutrition from the food her parents buy. From the butcher, they could buy grass fed beef steak. This would be expensive, but, according to one's tradition, it was justified on Friday evening or Sunday dinner. It would supply both omega 3 and omega 6 fatty acids, and it would be pure beef. And vegetables from the green grocer would be pure, unadulterated vegetables. The milk that would be delivered at her parents' door would be wholesome, balanced milk. The eggs, beans, and canned goods from the local grocer would be local eggs, tasty, and balanced in terms of fatty acids. But, then, if

---

193   Erasmus, Udo. Fats that Heal; Fats that Kill, 17th printing (2006), p.367.

this young girl grows up in the fifties, she would notice the replacement of local general grocers, green grocers, and butchers with supermarkets, with their own meat and produce sections. What she would probably not notice would be the development of factory farms and large commercial vegetable growers, which would use the supermarkets as their distribution agents for their factory farmed beef, poultry, or pork, as well as for the commercial vegetables. If she now got her food from supermarkets, she would be unaware that it was deficient in omega 3 fatty acids, several minerals, and over abundant in omega 6 fatty acids. And if she continued eating supermarket food through the fifties, sixties, and seventies, her body would slowly degenerate, for the over abundance of linoleic acid, for the lack of alpha-linolenic acid, for the antibiotics in the meat, and for the pathogens and pesticides in the vegetables. Then in 1981 her physiological degeneration would have attained the level of diagnoses of cardio-vascular disease and cancer. She would be disheartened. She had been afraid of such diagnoses, and here they came. But she couldn't be surprised. Her bridge partners, Milly and Susan, both have cancer. She guesses that it just happens. And if she retains sufficient curiosity to ask her physician how she could come to get cancer, he, with excellent medical training in pharmaceuticals and how to run offices, and with absolutely no training in dietetics, will tell her that he has no idea how it developed, that it just happens.

But with his ability to take an informative personal history, and with supermarket foods, particularly meats and vegetables, as blatant evidence, how could this physician be unaware? Well, with his personal commitment to be fully professional, it is not a case of willful ignorance, rather it is a case of institutional ignorance. It is a result of pharmaceutical industrial involvement in the medical school curriculum. It breeds medical training detrimental to effective medical practice, but it also helps guarantee profits for the pharmaceutical industry.

Speaking of the pharmaceutical industry, let us now discuss the pharmaceutical/medical method of treating breast cancer. First was the discovery that estrogen is related to breast cancer. As a research article, "Estrogen Brings Breast Cancer Back," reviewed on WebMD states:

Breast cancer survivors whose bodies make the least estrogen have the lowest chance of breast cancer recurrence as in those whose breast cancer did not come back.

Estrogen levels – measured soon after initial breast cancer treatment – were trice as high in women whose breast cancer returned as in those whose breast cancer did not come back.[194]

The women referred to in this study were nearly all post menopausal, which is about the time when most breast cancer is diagnosed. For more than 30 years it has been known that there is a relation of estrogen with breast cancer. At about that time ICI Pharmaceuticals developed tamoxifen. ICI Pharmaceuticals became AstraZeneca, and marketed tamoxifen under the trade names Nolvadex, Istubal, and Valodex. But even before the patent expired, the drug was widely referred to by its generic name, tamoxifen.[195]

Tamoxifen has been the main drug against breast cancer. But it does not cure breast cancer. It does not kill breast cancer cells. It, rather, "freezes" them; so, while the drug is administered they cannot reproduce. The way it works is that it is taken as a pill. It is transferred from the intestinal system to the liver, where it is metabolized into active metabolites, one of which is 4-hydroxytamoxifen. In breast tissue 4-hydroxytamoxifen acts as an estrogen receptor antagonist, thereby preventing the processing of estrogen. This prevents cancerous cells from dividing.

But if estrogen is the cause of breast cancer, then why does it mostly effect post-menapausal women? The age range when estrogen is most copiously produced by the woman's body is the late teens and early twenties. Then why does not breast cancer strike these women frequently? One response may be that the disease is diagnosed mostly in post-menapausal women, whose estrogen is non-ovarian (estrone). But there are women who are pre-menapausal, in the late thirties, early forties, who are stricken with breast cancer; so, if it is estrogen which causes breast cancer, and these pre-menapausal woman, producing estrogen in their ovaries (17beta-estradiol) get it, then why do not twenty year olds, who produce ovarian estrogen in spades? The short answer is that these young women, most of whom eat supermarket food from commercial farmers and factory farms, have not had enough time for their bodies to degenerate to the point of producing tumors, which may be diagnosed as breast cancer. By the time these women are in their late thirties and forties their bodies would have

---

194   http://www.webmd.com/breast-cancer/news/20080307/estrogen-brings-breast-cancer-back

195   http://en.wikipedia.org/wiki/Tamoxifen

degenerated sufficiently that one expression of this degeneration would be breast cancer.

So, breast cancer having been diagnosed, tamoxifen is prescribed. As we have already stated, this drug has the effect of freezing cancer cells in their proverbial tracks; it prevents them from reproducing. One effect, therefore, of tamoxifen is to stymie breast cancer. What other effects does tamoxifen have? Well, the American Cancer Society lists tamoxifen as a known carcinogen, for its increased risk of uterine cancer.[196] But the American Cancer Society also said that tamoxifen should still be used where the risk of breast cancer was larger than the risk of uterine cancer.

Another effect of tamoxifen is that it can cause a rapid increase in triglyceride concentration in the blood, thereby increasing the risk of clotting (thromboembolism), especially during and immediately after major surgery or periods of inactivity. The fourth effect is fatty liver, otherwise known as steatorrhoeic hepatosis or steatosis hepatis.[197] A fifth effect is the reduction of libido. The sixth effect, which is beneficial, is the prevention of osteoporosis.

Tamoxifen has been around for over 30 years, and much has been written about it. The risks it presents are also widely appreciated. But, despite these risks, if tamoxifen is stopped with a patient with breast cancer, the breast cancer cells will again divide and grow. Another factor is that there is a sharp discontinuation rate among women, particularly the younger cancer patients.

> The researchers found that at 12 months 22 percent of women had ceased using the drug. At 24 months 28 percent had stopped tamoxifen, and at 3.5 years 35 percent had stopped the treatment without commencing an alternative therapy.[198]

Most of the women who discontinued were noted to have started taking anti-depression drugs just prior to discontinuation of tamoxifen.

---

196   "Known and Probable Carcinogens," The American Cancer Society (2006-02-03), found in http://www.cancer.org/docroot/PED/cotent/PED_1_3x_Known_and_Probable_Carcinogens.asp?sitearea=PED

197   http://en.wikipedia.org/wiki/Tamoxifen

198   "Tamoxifen Discontinuation Rates Surprisingly High In Clinical Practice," in http://www.cancer.org/docroot/MED/content/MED_2_1x_Tamoxifen_Discontinuation_Rates_Surprisingly_High_In_Clinical_Practice.asp

So, another drug had to be used. The second most used drug for breast cancer is an aromatase inhibitor. Aromatase is an enzyme present in many cells, and it functions to catalyze the conversion of testosterone to estradiol, in the ovaries, and androstenedione to estrone, in the liver, the breasts, the adrenal glands, and some other cells. So, if aromatase can be inhibited, to the degree it is, that much estrogen is prevented from being developed.

Several aromatase inhibitors were developed. The predominant one is exemastane, with the trade name, Aromasin. This drug has been used in combination with tamoxifen, and, in recent years, has replaced tamoxifen after two or three years. As a steroidal drug, Aromasin can quickly migrate to every cell where it can be effective.

But, before it is prevented from developing, we should understand, in addition to promoting breast cancer, what estrogen does in the body. Well, it contributes to the maintenance of blood vessels and skin, in increases bone strength, it increases the liver production of binding proteins, it increases HDL and lowers LDL, and it promotes lung function by supporting alveoli.

Because of limitations of tamoxifen and exemastane, and their unhappy side effects, a new drug was introduced to treat breast cancer. This new drug is trastuzumab, marketed as Herceptin. This drug, developed by Genentech of San Francisco, is more elegant, in that it targets a specific molecule in the cell membrane. This molecule is HER2/neu, and is a growth factor. After puberty and the breasts have been fully developed, HER2/neu should be largely inactive. When HER2/neu is 'overexprssed,' very active, which it is in 15-20% of breast cancers, it is an unambiguous indicator of neoplasm, cancer. Trastuzemab (Herceptin) acts directly to neutralize, deactivate, HER2/neu.

There are two biological problems with trastuzemab. First, it has a low response rate. As many as 70% of breast cancer patients do not react. Second, resistance to it increases as it is administered. Further, a full treatment with trastuzemab costs between $60,000 and $70,000. If not covered by insurance, or without insurance, such costs are prohibitive for most people. Even if such costs are covered by insurance, the wide use of such drugs would greatly increase the costs of medical care.

So, the pharmaceutical/medical treatment of breast cancer necessarily also degenerates the body of the patient, or it is of limited use, and has a great cost. This is a terrible bind to be put it. Such treatment is correctly indicated for about .02% of women who have a genetic predisposition for cancer, as well as those women who have absorbed a high amount of pollutants, such as dioxin, into their system.

But for other women diagnosed with breast cancer, and that includes most, such costs are unnecessary, and all of this is unnecessary interference with the body, and superficial treatment of symptoms of the larger condition. A healthy woman, who is not among the small minority with a genetic predisposition and who has not contaminated herself with carcinogenic contaminants, does not get breast cancer. And a woman so contaminated can be analyzed as such, and analysis may also be possible to determine genetic determinacy. But a woman severely physically degenerated from the chronic deficiency in alpha-linolenic acid (omega 3) and its metabolites, a chronic oversupply of linoleic acid (omega 6 and its metabolites), as well as a deficiency in at least a couple of vitamins and a few or more of the nutritional minerals, will exhibit breast cancer, cardio vascular disease, depression, and several other symptoms of this degeneration. The proper treatment is not to swat at symptoms with drugs, but to supply the deficiencies and have the patient change her previous lifestyle in terms of eating and exercise.

So, an orthomolecular treatment would include a clinical dose of flax oil, accompanied by a sulphur containing protein food, such as cottage cheese, as well as other vitamins and/or dietary minerals which have been found in the diagnosis to be deficient. The administration of such treatment, with the commitment of the patient to henceforth include in her diet foods she had heretofore neglected, will result in the total elimination of the cancers, and the development of a body chemistry which will immunize her from cancer in the future. Of course, the specific treatment and prescription would depend on her diagnosis.

We have discussed breast cancer, the way it would be treated orthomolecularly and the way it would be treated pharmaceutically. Let us now turn to depression.

Approximately 14.4 million Americans suffer from clinical depression. But incidence does not fall evenly on the sexes. One in eight, or 12% of all women are depressed, but only 7% of men have been similarly diagnosed. So, it is a significant problem, and quite significant for woman.

Let's start with the pharmaceutical/medical approach. How does such a practitioner look upon depression? Well, he has to prescribe a drug. But might the depression be related to the patient's lifestyle?, to what she has been eating? Who knows? But the drug will take care of it.

There have been four general types of antidepressant drugs.[199]

- Trycyclic antidepressants (TCAs) These are some of the first antidepressants. They primarily inhibit the levels of two chemical messengers, norepinephrine and serotonin.

- Monoamine oxidase inhibitors (MAOIs) These are another early form of antidepressant. These drugs are most effective in people with depression who do not respond to other treatments. Substances in certain foods, such as cheese, beverages like wine, and medications can interact with an MAOI, so; people taking this medication must adhere to strict dietary restrictions. For this reason these antidepressants also aren't usually the first drugs used.

- Selective serotonin reuptake inhibitors (SSRIs) These are a newer form of antidepressant. These drugs work by increasing the amount of serotonin in the brain.

- Serotonin and norepinephrine reuptake inhibitors (SNRIs) These are another newer form of antidepressant. They treat depression by increasing the availability of serotonin and norepinephrine.

The first type of antidepressant drugs, the trycyclic antidepressants (TCA), are generally not used these days because of the additional, non-prescribed effects it has on the patient. These other effects are dry mouth, blurred vision, increased fatigue and sleepiness, weight gain, muscle tremors, constipation, bladder problems such as urine retention, dizziness, daytime drowsiness, increased heart rate, and sexual problems. The second type, Monoamine oxidase inhibitors (MAO) are also not used very much because of the diet restriction requirements as well as the non-prescribed effects, which include headache, heart racing, chest pain, neck stiffness, nausea and vomiting. The drug counsels patients to seek medical assistance immediately if such effects occur.

The most prescribed antidepressant drugs in 2007 are in Table 6 just below:

---

199 "Depression: Medication Options," from WebMed at http://www.webmd.com/depression/medication-options

Table 6
Top Depression Medications - 2007

	Medication	Used for	Prescriptions in U.S. 2007
1.	Lexapro	Depression, Anxiety	27,023,000
2.	Effexor XR	Depression, Anxiety	17,200,000
3.	Cymbalta	Depression	12,551,000
4.	Wellbutrin XL	Depression	6,370,000
5.	Budeprion* XL	Depression, Seasonal Affective Disorder	4,808,000
6.	Budeprion* SR	Depression	3,484,000
7.	Paxil CR	Depression	2,491,000
8.	Zoloft	Depression, Anxiety	1,615,000

* Budeprion is also known as Bupropion, and was previously known as Wellbutrin.

For 14.4 million clinically diagnosed cases of depression Table 6 indicates many prescriptions. The total for the top eight prescribed depression medications is 75,542,000. Of course the total prescriptions includes renewal prescriptions, and 5.2 renewals over the course of a year are not excessive.

All of the top depression medications listed are serotonin reuptake inhibitors. Wellbutrin, Effexor, and Cymbalta also increase the amount of norepinephrine in the brain; Wellbutrin also increases dopamine in the brain. In the brain, norepinephrine is a neurotransmitter which, acting as a stress hormone, it affects parts of the brain where attention and responding actions are controlled. Along with epinephrine, norepinephrine also underlies the fight-or-flight response, directly increasing heart rate, triggering the release of glucose from energy stores, and increasing blood flow to skeletal muscle. However, when norepinephrine is taken as a drug, its function is to increase blood flow by constricting the blood vessels, and triggering a reflex which drops the heart rate.[200]

The main function of dopamine is to inhibit the release of prolactin from the anterior lobe of the pituitary, thereby inhibiting lactation. Another

---

200   http://en.wikipedia.org/wiki/Norepinephrine

function it has is to inhibit the conditional response to a rewarding stimulus, and to help the brain determine a pattern of rewards.[201]

But the main target of depression drugs is serotonin, and depression drugs operate to either increase or decrease the amount of serotonin. All of the drugs listed above operate to increase serotonin. Serotonin is a neurotransmitter. In the brain it plays a role in the modulation of anger, aggression, body temperature, mood, sleep, sexuality, appetite, and metabolism. By increasing the amount of serotonin in the brain there will be changes in these responses and feelings. Now, consider, a person who has approached a physician, and who has received a prescription for one of these drugs is a person who is not happy, who feels sad, in fact, miserable, with, probably, reduced appetite and sexuality. Now she takes the drug, and it changes her moods. Well, any change from miserable is bound to be felt as positive. Given that the circumstances she is in have not changed, there may also be a tone of unreality in her feeling. But the drug does work.

So, this pharmaceutical intervention must be considered positively, should it not? Well, consider some other facts. The focus has been the operation of serotonin in the brain. But the drug increases the level of serotonin, generally. And 90% of the serotonin in a person's body is in that person's general intestines. It resides and operates within, what are called, enterochromaffin[202] cells which are part of the lining of the gastrointestinal tract. There the serotonin stimulates peristalsis.[203] Serotonin also occupies the platelets in the blood vessels, where it acts as vasoconstrictor, to stop bleeding. Thus, an excess of serotonin not only disrupt the digestive system, it can also cause hypertension, and initiate a syndrome of cardiac valve fibrosis.

As we have pointed out in the discussions of hypercholesterolemia and breast cancer, above, pharmaceutical drugs often, and in each of the three hypothetical cases discussed, disrupt many areas of the body in attempting to address the symptom, which pharmaceuticals call "disease." Often the disruption is more harmful to the patient than the symptom itself. And, in the case of depression, do any of the drugs listed serve to cure the patient of depression? Of course not; that is not what the pharmaceutical

---

201   http://en.wikipedia.org/wiki/Dopamine

202   Enterochromaffin is so called because "entero" refers to being in the intestinal tract, and "chromaffin" relates to fact that it shares the chromium salt reaction with the chromaffin cells of the adrenal glands.

203   http://en.wikipedia.org/wiki/Serotonin

mission is about . Pharmaceutical firms did not get wealthy curing people. And, quite opposite to curing, about 2.2 million people are injured by prescription drugs each year,[204] it is estimated that about 200,000 people annually in the United States die from adverse drug reactions.[205] It is very expensive, in terms of lives, the quality of life, and money, to maintain this pharmaceutical/medical system.

So, for a moment, let's put reality aside, and let imagination take central stage. And let's imagine, of a sudden, that all pharmaceutical firms disappeared! Major changes would quickly ensue. Within a week factory farms would cease operations. Putting animals in severely concentrated facilities is creating disease generations facilities. Without antibiotics, and huge quantities of them, these operations cannot continue. So, factory farms would also disappear. And, without factory farm manure, commercial farmers would find it difficult to fertilize their agricultural operations. Within three to twelve months, depending on what time during the year the pharmaceuticals suddenly disappeared, commercial farms would suffer decreases of production. Supermarkets would be hard pressed to get their usual deliveries of cheap beef, chicken, and pork, as well as of adequate supplies of commercial vegetables. They would have to seek out local or nearby suppliers of beef, chicken, and pork, and nearby suppliers of vegetables and fruits. These would be local farms raising grass fed cattle. Many of them also raise outdoor pigs, and chickens. A significant percentage of the truck farmers, the farmers raising vegetables, would be organic, or farmers which do not use herbicides and insecticides. So, simply by having all pharmaceutical firms disappear, within two years most of Americans, North Americans, will be healthier, and most of the degenerate symptoms will pass away. Goodness, what imagination can do! But it does give a clue about possible policies which would promote the health of Americans.

Getting back to reality, and as we have seen in discussing three quite different symptoms, "diseases," that pharmaceutical drugs are never designed to cure the patient. That is not what pharmaceuticals are about. But what do patients want from medical service? It is not a stretch to say that patients want to be rid of their malady; they want to be cured. There is

---

204 "Medical System is Leading Cause of Death and Injury in US," in http://www.newmediaexplorer.org/sepp/2003/10/29/medical_system_is_leading_cause_of_death_and_injury_in_us.htm

205 Fraser, Jessica. "Statistic Prove Prescription Drugs are 16,400% More Deadly Than Terrorists," in http://www.naturalnews.com/009278.html

no help from the pharmaceutical system. But the orthomolecular method may help a patient be cured. Let's now discuss how such treatment might occur.

First, if food allergies are suspected, a detailed food history may be taken, and the patient put on an elimination diet. Orthomolecularly, the following nutrients may be prescribed: alpha-linolenic acid (Omega 3), at two and one-half ounces or three tablespoons in the form of flax oil, and ascorbic acid (Vitamin C), 1,000 mg, to be consumed daily. Also, a comprehensive Vitamin B tablet containing zinc (Stress Formula), Vitamin D, at 1,000 mg daily, and selenium, calcium, and magnesium. Behaviorally, the patient should find a way, or be counseled, to remove herself from stress situations. The patient would also be strongly advised to exercise herself, by walking or a more vigorous activity, at least several times each week.

Of course, a particular treatment would be administered to each patient after careful diagnosis. The above only provides the general approach, for illustrative purposes. The described orthomolecular treatments for hypercholesterolemia and breast cancer were also only for illustrative purposes. A patient with one of those deficiency conditions, who seeks an orthomolecular practitioner, will receive a particular treatment relating to her diagnosis.

9 – Agriculture and Water Conservation for the Twenty First Century

THE ONLY WAY CORN and soybeans can be profitably grown on the Great Plains is with the use of artificial fertilizers and the drawing of water from the Ogallala Aquifer. The artificial fertilizers are so copiously applied that there is usually runoff of fertilizer into the streams and rivers, polluting them as well as the large, increasing dead zone in the Gulf of Mexico. Drawing water out of the Ogallala Aquifer for agriculture speeds up the depletion of that large aquifer, jeopardizing the water supply for the cities which depend on it.

Of the eight states, or parts of states, that lie over the Ogallala Aquifer, at least 27 cities draw water from surface waters, or near surface aquifers, which contribute to the Ogallala Aquifer, or draw directly from the Ogallala Aquifer. New Mexico and northern Texas, desert areas, draw directly from the Ogallala Aquifer. The cities in these areas which draw directly from the Ogallala Aquifer are Amarillo and Lubbock, both in the Texas "pan handle," and Albuquerque and Clovis, both in New Mexico. The major cities in eastern Colorado, South Dakota, Kansas, Oklahoma, Nebraska, and eastern Wyoming all drew from surface water, or near surface aquifers related to surface water. These water sources, however, directly over the Ogallala Aquifer, all contribute to that Aquifer.

All of these cities, including Albuquerque, Clovis, Lubbock, and Amarillo, use less water than does agriculture, and they, therefore, deplete the Aquifer more slowly. As the Ogallala Aquifer replenishes very slowly, the four cities which draw directly from it ought to find alternative sources of water. Playas, a dry lake bed for most of the year, filling, or partially filling, with water in the winter, the wet season, in the southern Ogallala Aquifer land area are areas which absorb water for transit to the Ogallala Aquifer. Some of these playas have been destroyed by farming or development. Because much of the area of the land covering the Ogallala Aquifer is covered with water impermeable caliche, calcium carbonate, the destruction of the playas decreases the Aquifers very slow replenishment rate. It is irresponsible to reduce the replenishment rate, and there is no justification for it.

It is also exceedingly irresponsible to grow corn, and other field crops, on the land above the Ogallala Aquifer, with water drawn from that aquifer, and using artificial fertilizer and pesticides, much of which runs off onto the delicate Great Plains prairie land. The runoff enters surface rivers which are in the Mississippi River watershed. These waters collect in rivers used by several cities, before it goes down the Mississippi to contribute to the dead area of the Gulf of Mexico. Why the draining of the Ogallala Aquifer, to irrigate fields which pollute waters far and wide, to produce crops contaminated with insecticide is even tolerated is a question that needs to be answered.

To reiterate, we are each made of the food, air, and water we take in, or which our mother took in. And, in terms of food, we are evolutionarily leaf, fruit, vegetable, root, and nut eaters, with occasional meat, mostly from grass eating antelopes. So, we should abandon the draining of the Ogallala aquifer for the growing of corn, for all agriculture, and let the prairie revert to grassland, feeding a growing buffalo herd. This could be selectively harvested for meat.

It should be obvious by now that it is immoral as well as irresponsible to continue the three billion dollar subsidy for corn, which overproduces corn, depletes the Ogallala Aquifer, pollutes waterways far and wide, and is primarily used to sustain a factory farm system, which produces no healthy beef, no healthy chicken, no healthy pork, and no healthy eggs and milk, and is responsible for most of the disease in the most diseased nation in the world. If some demon were to divert three billions of public money to undermine the health and safety of America, he couldn't do it better than Congress has with its three billion dollar corn subsidy.

That subsidy could be better used to defray the costs of desalination plants on the shores of the Gulf of Mexico, as well as on the Pacific, and on the Atlantic. The Federal Government could then subsidize the construction of a water pipeline to New Mexico and northern Texas. In the northern states the Federal Government could subsidize the construction of large green houses, and local solar and wind electrical generation systems to provide light and heat to the green houses. Rather than destroying the health of the American people, the government could use subsidies to build the infrastructure for healthy food and a healthy American population.

10 - The Restoration
of National Health

THE RESTORATION OF NATIONAL health would have many benefits, in addition to improving the feelings, vitality, and outlook of the American adult population. It would provide more workers for our industries and new agricultural production. It would drastically reduce health costs in America, by about 70% to 80%. It would increase the general wealth of the country, and it would, perforce, reduce the pollution of waterways. It would also restore the natural health of the Great Plains.

This restoration would require Congress to cease playing politics, in the crudest sense of the word, and start responding to public needs in terms of health, water, and safety. It would require the federal government, for a change, to assiduously abide by the law. It would require the federal government, for the health and safety of the American people, whom it exists to serve, to pass new laws governing the use of insecticides and chemical fertilizer, as well a stipulating what would constitute a comprehensive, health providing, chemical fertilizer.

But mostly, the federal government has to simply administer laws it already has on the books, which, by the President's oath of office, it is supposed to administer. Clean, navigable interstate waters require that the watersheds of those streams, as well as of all contributing streams, have to be free of pollution and obstruction. You don't have to be a nuclear physicist to understand this. Any stream is made up of all of the streams that come to it. The cleanliness and purity of any stream depends on the cleanliness and purity of all the streams that come to it. At least one

Supreme Court decision in this area, which did not evidence understanding of this, Rapanos v. United States, 547 U.S. 715 (2006), will have to be overridden.

And clean air means not only that there be a severe limit on the amount of methylmercury, emitted from coal fired electrical generators, in the air, as well as other molecules poisonous to breath in, but also substances which are extremely offensive to smell. It also means the limitation of carbon dioxide (CO^2) and methane (CH^4) in the atmosphere, which traps infrared radiation (heat) from escaping into space, thereby reducing the water and water vapor on the surface of the land. The major reason for the increase in CO^2 has been the oxidation of fossil fuels. The Environmental Protection Agency (EPA) has the authority to limit these emissions. Most of these emissions, of CO^2, come from vehicular traffic and coal fired electricity generators. The EPA also has the authority to limit the emission of chlorinated fluorocarbons (CFCs), which have much slower decay rates than carbon dioxide or methane.

With respect to the FDA, it is legally responsible for the safety regulation of food items. Partially hydrogenated oils in margarine and shortening contain transfats and are unsafe to eat. The FDA, consistent with its explicit legal responsibilities, should ban these items from sale as food. Furthermore, any reasonable definition of food must require that an item contain at least one nutritive substance. Most of the heat processed and heavily filtered oils one finds on supermarket shelves lack this qualification. They should not be sold as food. And the United States Department of Agriculture Food Safety and Inspection Service, which has the authority to regulate the meat of domestic animals, should ban the sale of feed lot cattle, infected with E-Coli 0157:H7, as unsafe. It is not an appropriate response that this beef can be irradiated with intense, focused beams of X-rays, or with highly basic ammonia. This form of irradiation destroys most of the nutrients in the meat, and the ammonia is unhealthy for human digestive systems. What is the point of eating meat devoid of nutrients, or unsafe?

The restoration of national health will require that the FDA fully honor its legal responsibilities. As for Congress, the single, most important contribution to national health it can do, is to eliminate the three billion dollar subsidy for corn. Zero it out. This is the financial sustenance of the most unhealthy food production system the country, the world, has ever known. It is hard to imagine that members of Congress understood that their support of the corn subsidy was undermining the health of the American people. It is more likely that they never considered the health and social consequences of this, or any subsidy. This is irresponsible, and each member of Congress who ever supported this corn subsidy shares the responsibility for millions of people suffering from deficiency diseases, and millions of premature deaths.

The ending of the corn subsidy will cause a fairly rapid reduction in the amount of corn grown, and the correlative rise in the price of corn. This will probably result in the decommissioning of a number of smaller feedlots. The larger feedlots may have to switch to hay and straw, as is done in European feedlots. If the feed were switched to hay and straw, the E-coli 0157:H7 problem will be eliminated. Irradiation will be unnecessary. This will improve the health of the beef as food. Of course the time required for the cattle to attain full weight for slaughter will be lengthened. This will increase the cost of beef. This, in turn, will reduce the amount of beef the average person, family, consumes. This will have the health dividend, by limiting the amount of meat people eat, which always has some cholesterol. Also the feedlot beef will still have some toxins. The increased cost of corn will probably also have beneficial effects on the factory chicken and pig farms.

If the federal government and Congress wanted to hasten the decline of the factory farms, and do something beneficial for the health of all Americans, they could legislate a tax on the sale of antibiotics. Even a minor tax would have major ramification for the factory farms, which use tons of antibiotics. A more substantial tax would decrease the use of antibiotics among the general public, which would decrease the spread of antibiotic resistant pathogens.

If Congress were also to legislate a tax on the sale of insecticides, this would decrease their use. The field products would be that much healthier, it would decrease the spread of insecticide resistant pests. Of course commercial farmer will have to re-learn the rotation of crops, and they will have to hire people to help them weed. They are clearly capable of doing that.

With the enactment of a regulatory tax on antibiotics and one on insecticides, with the elimination of the corn subsidy, we would begin to dismantle the poison generation system in this country, which has been masquerading as a food production system. And, with the FDA faithfully administering its enabling act, which is the Food, Drug and Cosmetic Act, also called Title 21, Chapter 9 of the United States Code,[206] with explicit authority to regulate food safety, it would ban the sale of partially hydrogenated oils, sold as margarine and shortening. The federal government could then also require the re-labeling of all refined, heat processed vegetable oils, which are devoid of nutrients, and cannot be referred to as food. We would still have carbonized soft drinks, with copious calories[207] and few nutrients, as well as white flour and white rice, and severely sweetened breakfast cereals. But, if we can reduce the use of antibiotics and insecticides, and correctly label or remove from the shelves, margarine and shortening made from partially hydrogenated oils, and refined, heat treated vegetable oils, we will significantly improve the health prospects for many, many people.

The absence of the corn subsidy will also probably reduce the number of farms, of acres, of corn grown over the Ogallala Aquifer. This will reduce toxic runoff in the Mississippi watershed.

People also need real oil for their health. Of course, after the elimination of the 'long shelf life,' very refined, filtered, heat treated oils, there will still be Virgin or Extra Virgin Olive Oil on the supermarket shelves. This is a good oil, but it is not sufficient for human health. Humans need oils which represent both Omega 3 and Omega 6 fatty acids. A balance of these will help digestion, skin tone, and guarantee good health. Such oils can be pressed from flax seeds, sunflower seeds, and hemp seeds. But for the oils to be healthy, they have to be unrefined, unfiltered, and packaged in small, opaque bottles which will have to be refrigerated, with expiration dates on each. People are accustomed to having eggs and milk which are perishable, and have expiration dates. They will have no difficulty in adjusting to perishable oils with expiration dates.

---

206   Which can be seen in http://www.fda.gov/opacom/laws/fdcact/fdctoc.htm

207   Technically, these are kilocalories. A calorie refers to the raising of one gram of water one degree Celsius. That is not much energy. So, generally, people are referring to the energy of raising one kilogram of water one degree Celsius. When it is said that a 145 pound person needs 2,000 calories daily for weight maintenance, reference is to kilocalories. But, in popular language, the term 'calorie' is used for 'kilocalorie,' and we will continue that usage.

Reference was made to hemp seeds in the preceding paragraph. Particularly what was referred to is industrial hemp, which has a long history among humanity and in this country, but which is not cultivated anymore in the United States. The reason its cultivation was discontinued involves many reasons other than intelligence or responsibility, and it involves one of the most severe pollution episodes in the history of humankind. We will digress to discuss that, but first we must digress to discuss the history of hemp cultivation in the world and in the United States.

Between the bark and inner, woody area, of the hemp plant are long, soft fibers, ideal for the making of cloth, ropes, and strong paper. These fibers are white, and do not need to be bleached for paper. If any whitening is required, hydrogen peroxide is all that is needed. It is a plant which does not leach the soil, and fairly resistant to pests; so, insecticide is not needed.

In China cloth was made from hemp at about 8,000 BCE. Between 4,500 and 2,800 BCE China made rope from hemp. The process to make paper from hemp was developed just over 2,000 years ago. The Chinese regarded its development as something they wanted to keep secret from others. It wasn't until 1,150 CE that Muslims in Europe started Europe's first hemp paper mill. For the next 850 years most paper was made from hemp fibers.

In the ensuing years, with the development of oceanic ships, hemp was important for providing canvas[208] for sails, and line (rope). During the years of transoceanic discovery and of oceanic battles, the lines and sails of all the ships were made from hemp.

Hemp was brought to America early in European colonization. It continued to be the source of paper and cloth, as well as canvas and ship line. The first two drafts of the Declaration of Independence were drafted on hemp paper. George Washington and Thomas Jefferson were hemp farmers. Benjamin Franklin owned a mill that made hemp paper.[209] Newspapers, Bibles, farmers' almanacs, school readers, stationery, all paper for printing or writing was made from hemp.

The seeds were used for food, and they were also pressed for oil. The oil was used in lamps, and for machinery. Rudolph Diesel designed his engine

---

208   'Canvas' is a vulgarization of the Latin word for hemp, which is 'cannibis.'

209   Much of this history is from a document of the North American Industrial Hemp Council, Inc., and can be accessed at http://naihc.org/hemp_information/hemp_facts.html

to run on hemp oil. Hemp oil, along with linseed (flax) oil, was also used in paints, resins, shellacs, and varnishes.

We now know that this oil, hemp oil, is very important for the human diet. It has both essential fatty acids, and in good proportion. Of course, this was not known before the Second World War.

But hemp is now not used for paper in the United States. Why? It is a friendly plant to the ecology, not leaching the soil. It is easily grown in most parts of the United States. An acre of hemp plants absorbs more atmospheric carbon than an acre of any species of tree, or an acre of mixed species of trees. Paper from hemp does not require that there be any deforestation, in the Amazon or in this country. The processing of hemp for paper does not require the use of chloride, which forms the widespread, carcinogenic polychorinated dibenzodioxin, popularly known as dioxin. And hemp can be used to make fabric of many sorts, including canvass, rope, plastic, and building materials for homes and other buildings. Finally, hemp seed produce a very nutritious oil for people.

Part of the reason has to do with the fact that industrial hemp is easily grown in most parts of the United States. How could DuPont, Dow, and Monsanto control that? The obvious answer is that they cannot. But they can, just like the pharmaceutical firms, control a process by patenting it, a process which breaks down wood to make paper. So, by licensing, these three firms control the entire paper making process. This allows them to make a lot of money. But wait one moment. How did the chemical firms get to control this process, given that paper making was wide spread, and industrial hemp production was nationwide? Ah, now begins the story. It is a story of mendacity and irresponsibility, writ large. It also involves the international pollution of air, water, and vegetables of a carcinogenic substance, and the dereliction of the United States Congress and Government.

Between 1916 and 1937 William Randolph Hearst engaged in 'journalism' which took leave of facts, and was dedicated to a policy goal. This has been called yellow journalism, and the Hearst newspapers were dedicated to confusing the distinction between the historic industrial hemp and the Mexican variety, which was recently being brought to the United States by Mexican immigrants. The Mexican term for hemp was marijuana. What Hearst was attempting to do, and was evidently successful, except for the industrial hemp growers, was to have people identify all hemp as marijuana. The motivation of Hearst to engage in this yellow journalism was to reduce competition for wood pulp paper, which he used for his newspapers. This was profitable for Hearst because he had extensive holding of forest land, and was heavily invested in wood pulp paper factories.[210]

The Hearst campaign grew in fervor after George W. Schlichten patented a new machine in 1917 for separating the fiber from the internal woody core ("hurds") of hemp stalks, reducing labor costs by over 90% and increasing fiber yield by 600%. That, combined with new technology to fashion paper and plastics from hemp-derived cellulose, gradually breathed new life into the hemp industry.[211] Hearst was determined to destroy that industry before its capabilities developed and become apparent.

During the Hoover administration Hearst was friendly with Andrew Mellon, Secretary of the Treasury. Because police powers are, constitutionally, reserved to the states, the federal government resorted to the use of its taxing powers to regulate narcotics, which, under the Harrison Act of 1914, were used to regulate morphine and cocaine. So, the Treasury Secretary was in charge of federal drug regulation. The specific office in the Treasury responsible for administering the Harrison Act was the Federal Bureau of Narcotics, headed by a commissioner. In 1931, Mellon appointed his niece's husband, Harry J. Anslinger, to be Commissioner of the Federal Bureau of Narcotics.

Hearst, a friend of Pierre DuPont, who shared oil interests with Andrew Mellon, received support for an aggressive campaign. A number of movies were made, including those with the titles: "Marijuana: Assassin of Youth," Devil's Weed," and "Reefer Madness." Hearst reported on these movies, and, constantly confusing industrial hemp with marijuana, reported *stories* about insanity and murders inspired by smoking marijuana.

As 1937 began, DuPont began preparing applications for patents for a chemical process to render wood pulp to paper making, and for processes to make plastics from oil. Then, DuPont learned that International Harvester, early in 1937, was manufacturing a machine, based on the process invented

---

210   Information for this story comes from a variety of sources. Some are: http://supak.com/hemp/hemp.htm and http://www.hemphasis.net/History/history.htm

211   From "The Chronology of Hemp Throughout History," at http://www.hemphasis.net/History/history.htm http://www.hemphasis.net/History/history.htm

by George W. Schlichten, which separated the pulp from the wood in hemp and which could process three tons of hemp an hour and produce higher quality fiber with less loss than wood-based pulp. Hemp was nearly ready to begin undercutting competing products. Popular Mechanics predicted that hemp would become America's first "billion dollar crop." It pointed out that "10,000 acres devoted to hemp will produce as much paper as 40,000 acres of average [forest] pulp land."[212]

This machine was also very promising, because it could enable hemp paper to be cost effective against the newly arising wood pulp paper. This was welcomed because wood pulp paper has shorter fiber strands than does hemp paper, and it has stiffer fiber. This results in wood pulp paper being harder and easier to tear, and it also does not have the longevity of hemp paper. Galileo's notes on his telescopic observations were written on hemp paper, and they still survive, and are quite readable. Even in the first decade of the twenty first century, Kimberly Clark, an American company, has a mill in France which produces hemp paper preferred for bibles because it lasts a long time and doesn't yellow.[213] But in 1937 the new mechanical method of scutching, separating the pulp from the woody section of the hemp stalk, developed by International Harvester and two other companies,[214] made hemp paper a promising industry for the twentieth century.

This panicked DuPont and Hearst, and they used all the leverage they had to get a bill passed in Congress, which was prepared and submitted by Harry J. Anslinger, and was signed into law by the President that same year. It was called The Marijuana Tax Act. The Act identified the plant whose cultivation was to be taxed as *Cannabis sativa*. Marijuana is of the same species as hemp, which DuPont and Hearst quite evidently knew. These are two of the varieties of *Cannabis sativa*, a member of the Mulberry family,[215] which has hundreds of varieties. Marijuana has been bred to have broad leaves which a content of delta 9 tetrahydrocannabinol (THC) between 3% and 20%. Industrial hemp has narrow leaves; it was bred for its stalks. Industrial hemp leaves have a THC content of between 0.05 and

212   http://unquietmind.com/revolt4.html

213   http://naihc.org/hemp_information/hemp_facts.html

214   http://unquietmind.com/revolt4.html

215   Lewin, Menachem, Pearce, Eli M. Handbook of Fiber Chemistry, (Marcel Dekker, 1998), p. 522.

1% .[216] There was no valid public policy reason to combine these varieties under the same regulation.

In 1969 the 1937 Marijuana Tax Act was found unconstitutional. And although the Act was suspended during the Second World War, when hemp was needed to make hawsers, a large rope used for the towing and mooring of ships, used by the U.S. Marines, and was found in violation of the Fifth Amendment in 1969, its provisions were, essentially, included in the Comprehensive Drug Abuse Prevention and Control Act of 1970.[217] The inclusion of industrial hemp in such an act is a legacy of the yellow journalistic campaign of Hearst in the 1920s and 1930s.

And there is one more thing about making paper from wood. Unlike hemp or kenaf or flax, wood has a fairly rigid fiber. It does, after all, have to support a 40 to 100 foot high tree. The DuPont process for making such fiber suitable for paper making had to use harsh chemicals. What it did was to process the wood pulp under heat with chlorine containing substances, to bleach the fiber in the process. Under heat, chlorine converts to polychlorinated dibenzodioxins, which have come to be known popularly as dioxins. Dioxins have a fairly rigid chemical structure, and are hydrophobic and lipidphilic. As it would ensconce itself in fats, with no normal bodily function, it was carcinogenic. In the paper making process, dioxins, as a waste product, were dumped in a nearby river used for cooling. Dioxins, as part of the bleaching process, also remained in the finished, bleached papers. Thus, in the rivers, dioxins would migrate to nearby fish. And paper put in the trash would be incinerated by municipalities, thereby releasing dioxins into the atmosphere. Because dioxins are carcinogenic, and because the number of cancer displaying dioxins dramatically increased, along with young children being impaired from nursing at the breast, the EPA strove to identify the source of such harmful pollution.

In 1987 the EPA identified and measured the dioxin emerging from incinerators. It found that incinerators accounted for 80% of the known dioxin levels. The EPA then required that a filter for dioxin be instituted. The most common method of converting dioxins was to pass the smoke which contained the dioxin through a high temperature (400°C) segment in the stack. As a result of the EPA emissions regulation over 90% of the incinerator emitted dioxins were reduced.[218]

---

216   http://naihc.org/hemp_information/hemp_facts.html

217   http://en.wikipedia.org/wiki/Marijuana_Tax_Act

218   http://www.hemphasis.net/Paper/paper_files/hempvtree.htm

Two years later the EPA discovered the origin of the dioxin pollution to be in tree pulp paper mills. It now became clear that the high temperature elemental chloride bleaching produced polychlorinated dibenzodioxins. Negotiations ensued to replace the use of elemental chloride with another method. Nine years later, in 2008, 80% of the wood pulp paper mills had converted to a non-dioxin producing process. Twenty percent of the wood paper mills in the United States in 2008 were still spewing dioxin.

The volume has been decreasing, but dioxins have spread to many waterways in the United States, and, airborne, have spread throughout Canada to the arctic north. People ingest dioxins by eating fish, beef, chicken, pork, cheese, and many vegetables and fruits. Probably a majority of the people in North America, in 2008, had at least some dioxin in their bodies.

For a new carcinogen, for which toxicologists and chemists had no historical knowledge, it was not unreasonable for the chemists in the EPA to take 19 years to discover the origin of the dioxin pollution. They were not aware of the wood pulp bleaching process. But the chemists in DuPont, and other chemical companies making the chemicals for the process can be assumed to have been aware. They can also be assumed to have been aware of the production of polychlorinated dibenzodioxins as a by product of the process. Yet none of them ever reported the dioxins to state health authorities or to the federal government. But why would they not? Well, one reason is that it threatened to significantly increase the cost of the wood pulp paper process.[219] This may well put mills out of business, thereby losing customers for DuPont. And so, dioxins aggregated, in the waterways, into fish, and in the air, into everything else, until the EPA discovered the origin of dioxin pollution.

This too, is part of the system of the poisoning of Americans. It consists of a decision by the United States Congress and Government to ban the use of hemp for paper, and other products, including plastics, and to use wood primarily. A high level of dioxins in one's body will produce cancer, and cancer thus produced cannot be cured orthomolecularly. The *foreign* shape of a dioxin molecule, and its strong lipidphilicity, prevents any enzyme from attaching to it and removing it. As has been said above, a diagnosed disease can be the result of a deficiency of one or more essential nutrients, a pathogen, or from pollution. With respect to the United States government commitment to wood pulp paper, people were poisoned by

---

219 http://www.wipo.int/pctdb/en/wo.jsp?IA=WO1994025669&wo=199402566 9&DISPLAY=DESC

the pollutant dioxin, which resulted in the incapacitation and death of a significant number.

One must conclude that the reason wood pulp paper was favored over hemp, although it has reduced our forests and produced inferior paper, is greed. Greed for individual gain, which ignores and is opposed to the people's interest and health, and, in fact, has been responsible for thousands of cancer deaths. Allowed to go unregulated, such greed can undermine people's health and, in the longer term, disintegrate civilization. So, it is important for the federal government, for Congress, to supervise and regulate all chemical, drug, food production and delivery, vehicle, and appliance manufacturers. Who else can check greed? Who else has the capacity to do so? But for Congress and the federal government to do so it has to, consistent with the oath of office each member, requires it to commit itself to the law and the public interest. It is not acting in the public interest to support a corn subsidy which sickens half the people, and prematurely kills about 500,000 each year. Nor is it in the public interest to maintain a ban on the cultivation of hemp, in favor of deforesting the country, polluting most of North America with a severe carcinogenic substance, and producing inferior paper.

But why should Congress favor a paper making system which deforests the country, which spews pollution far and wide, and which, in the end, makes an inferior type of paper, instead of allowing the cultivation of hemp, which does not exhaust resources, which employs more people, and which produces a finer quality of paper? This does not seem to be a rational policy. A number of people say they are opposed to the cultivation and use of marijuana. That may be, and there are a number of reasons to oppose the cultivation and use of marijuana, but that has nothing to do with the cultivation of hemp. Police say that they cannot distinguish industrial hemp from marijuana with an infrared detector. Since industrial hemp and marijuana are not grown in the same places, this does not seem logical. Quantity and location would seem to afford a distinction. It is unlikely that it would be marijuana on 600 acres of North Dakota. So, it doesn't seem to be a valid argument. In any event, the police would have to arrive on site to pursue the matter. I'm sure the North Dakota hemp farmer would offer them some coffee.

Yet another reason for the cultivation of hemp is provide plentiful, and therefore inexpensive, hemp oil for the food market. If there were a great quantity of hemp cultivated, filtered hemp oil could also be used to power diesel engines; thus, removing them from the dwindling petroleum market.

Hemp oil could also replace the kerosene based fuel for lanterns. But in a healthy society, unrefined, mechanically pressed hemp oil is an important source of both essential omega fatty acids, both Omega 3 and Omega 6. Since hemp cultivation would be distributed across the country, this would afford the delivery of fresh hemp oil to local markets, and filtered hemp oil for diesel engines in cars, trucks, and diesel-electric locomotives.

So, a healthy America would have to limit the use of antibiotics and insecticides. It would have to be absolutely intolerant of any operation which issued pollutants. It would have local or regional farms which could deliver fresh vegetables and fruits, which haven't been subjected to insecticides. People would have to return to seasonal eating. However, if a company, individuals, or the government were to invest in large, anaerobic, nitrogen filled, storage facilities, fruits and vegetables, without refrigeration, could be preserved without spoilage, for the winter and spring months. This would allow us to have foods year round, without having to transport them three or twelve thousand miles.

For those who wish to eat meat, the elimination of the corn subsidy will turn many cattle farmers back to pasture raising of cattle. The number of grass fed cattle should increase throughout the country. There may be fewer cattle, but most of these will be grass fed. People also will have learned that they should limit the amount of meat they have in their diet. An increased price for beef may do that, but it is essential that people understand the need to limit meat to ensure a well balanced diet.

So, we have the ability as a country, if we are willing to take action, to eliminate the current system of poisoning, of manifestly unhealthy food, and substitute it with a system of fresh, healthy food for all. But systems have inertia, and, in the case of the United States, strong vested interests whose interest they believe, in their perverted minds, is to maintain the current disease producing system. Thus, as has already been advised, individuals who wish to maintain their health will have to seek out local, preferably organic, farmers and their distribution agencies, food cooperatives or farmers' markets. And for those who need to use supermarkets, beware of unpackaged foods, and, for packaged foods, carefully read the ingredients. There are web sites identified above for those who want to purchase safe meat, if grass fed meat is not available locally. Until enough people become aware of the current atrocity of producing meat and vegetables in this country, sufficient to change it, individuals and families can have a healthy diet with just a little extra effort.

Glossary

AEROBIC

Aerobic is an adjective which means requiring air, usually oxygen. It is commonly used to describe those organisms which rely on the intake of oxygen in order to live, specifically, in order to oxidize nutrients. This is in contradistinction to organisms, such as those in the mid-oceanic trenches, or the bacteria in the human intestines, which do not use oxygen.

AMINO ACID

There are 20 standard amino acids which are either used to synthesize proteins and other biomolecules or oxidized to urea and carbon dioxide as a source of energy. Thus, the amino acids are the basic components of proteins and other molecules in the body.

ANAEROBIC

Anaerobic organisms, most commonly bacteria, either survive only in environments without oxygen, or in environments with a low density of oxygen. These bacteria metabolize usually with fermentation, or by reducing iron, manganese, nitrates, mercury, or sulfates. Though these bacteria can survive by these anaerobic means, the efficiency of their metabolism is far less than aerobic bacteria.

The intestinal bacterial colony in each human is anaerobic.

ANION

An anion is a negatively charged ion. An ion is an atom or a molecule which has gained or lost one or more valence electrons. If an ion has gained one or more electrons, and, consequently, has more electrons than protons, it is referred to as a anion.

ANTIBIOTIC

Despite its name, an antibiotic, meaning against all microorganisms, current human antibiotics are antibacterial only. They use naturally occurring compounds, and they work by attacking the cell wall, a structure peculiar to bacteria. As the human system incorporates symbiotic bacteria, antibiotics can be used against human pathogens, but can also be threat to the human system. Chronic, repeated use of antibiotics has also spawned a number of antibiotic resistant bacteria.

AQUIFER

An aquifer is a subterranean body of water. Some aquifers are near the surface of the land, others are deeper in the earth. Aquifers exist among porous rock, or unconsolidated substances, such as sand, gravel, silt, or clay. The Ogallala Aquifer in the United States contains fossil water, from the last glaciation, or before. It is being drained for agriculture or civic use at a rate nine times its replenishment rate.

ARRHYTHMIA

Cardiac arrhythmia, also referred to as dysrhythmia, is a term for any of a large and heterogeneous group of conditions in which there is abnormal electrical activity in the heart. The heart beat may be too fast or too slow, and may be regular or irregular. Some arrhythmia are life-threatening medical emergencies that can result in cardiac arrest and sudden death. Others cause aggravating symptoms such as an abnormal awareness of heart beat (palpitations), and may be merely annoying. Others may not be associated with any symptoms at all, but pre-dispose toward potentially life threatening stroke or embolus. And some arrhythmia are very minor and can be regarded as normal variants. In fact, most people will sometimes feel their heart skip a beat, or give an occasional extra strong beat, neither of which is usually a cause for alarm.

ATHEROSCLEROSIS

Atherosclerosis is a disease affecting arterial blood vessels. It results from the increased stickiness of plaques in the artery, and the deposition of a great quantity of small particle low density lipoproteins (LDL). When the high density lipoproteins (HDL) are unable to remove the LDL particles from the macrophage white blood cells, these latter accumulate and cause inflammation, another component of atherosclerosis.

AUTOIMMUNE

Autoimmunity is the failure of a person's immune system to recognize its own body. This produces attacks of the immune system on its own body. The diseases related to this aberrant immune system operation are rheumatoid arthritis, Celiac disease, lupus, and type 1 diabetes.

BACTERIA

Bacteria are unicellular micro-organisms which lack a nucleus. They have a large variety of shapes, ranging from spheres to rods to spirals. Although very small, bacteria are very numerous. In the human body, there are ten times the number of bacterial cells as there are human cells. Except for some ingested pathogens, or pathogens on the surface of the skin, bacteria in the human body are part of the humans system. They process ingested food and transfer nutrients to the rest of the body. They inhabit joints, allowing the joint's lubricated motion.

BIOACTIVE

Bioactive compounds are compounds which play a regulatory role to reduce inflammation by inhibiting the transport of inflammatory agents to a site. Bioactive compounds are, therefore, said to be immunoregulatory.

BIOMASS

Biomass is the mass of all of the living organisms in a category, such as the biomass of algae, bacteria, or multicellular animals. The term also refers to the biological material which can be used for fuel or industrial material.

BI-POLAR SYNDROME

Bi-polar syndrome, usually referred to as the bi-polar disorder, is a psychological disorder characterized by experiencing two opposing moods, an unusually elevated mood, mania, and depression. These may be separated by periods of normal behavior.

CALICHE

Caliche is a hardened deposit of calcium carbonate. This calcium carbonate cements together other materials, including gravel, sand, clay, and silt. Caliche occurs worldwide, generally in arid or semi-arid regions, including in central and western Australia, in the Kalahari Desert, in the High Plains of the western USA, and in the Sonoran Desert. Caliche is also known as hardpan, calcrete, kankar (in India), or duricrust. The term caliche is Spanish and is originally from the Latin calx, meaning lime.

CAMPYLOBACTER

The term Campylobacter, meaning "twisted bacteria," is the name of a genus of curved, rod shaped bacteria. Technically, they are gram-negative, spiral, microaerophilic bacteria. At least a dozen species of this genus have been implicated in human diseases, the most common being Campylobacter jejeuni, and Campylobacter coli. In recent years, these bacteria commonly derive from factory farms, and are typically acquired by humans by the eating of meats derived from these factory farms.

CATION

A cation is a positively charged ion. An ion is an atom or a molecule which has gained or lost one or more valence electrons. If an ion has lost one or more electrons, and, consequently, has more protons than electrons, it is referred to as a cation.

COCCIDIOSIS

Coccidia are macroscopic protozoa parasites. They are obligate, intracellular parasites, which means that they must live and reproduce within an animal cell. These parasites are animal species specific, and are acquired, usually, by the ingesting of feces. These parasites are common among factory farm animals.

COMMENSAL

In ecology, commensalism is a kind of symbiotic relationship between two organisms where one benefits and the other is not significantly harmed or helped (like a bird living in a tree). Some scientists–biologists, physiologists– use this term to describe the relationship of the bacteria colonies in the human intestines and skin. Others refer to the relationship as far more mutualistic, as genuine symbiosis.

CYTOCHROME OXIDASE

Cytochrome oxidase is a large transmembrane molecule complex found in mitochondria and in bacteria. It is involved in the last stage of cellular respiration, and is a component of the ATP forming operation.

DOCOSANOIDS

Docosanoids are signaling molecules made by oxygenation of twenty-two-carbon essential fatty acids, (EFAs), especially Docosahexaenoic acid (DHA), which is derived from α-linolenic acid (Omega 3 fatty acid).

DOCOSATRIENES

Docosanoids include docosatrienes and resolvins. Docosatrienes and resolvins are highly potent neuroprotectors and are anti-inflammatory.

EICOSANOIDS

Eicosanoids are signaling molecules made by oxygenation of twenty-carbon essential fatty acids, (EFAs). They exert complex control over many bodily systems, mainly in inflammation or immunity, and as messengers in the central nervous system. The networks of controls that depend upon eicosanoids are among the most complex in the human body. Eicosanoids derive from both Omega 3 and Omega 6 fatty acids. Those deriving from linoleic acid (Omega 6) are generally inflammatory. Those deriving from α-linolenic acid (Omega 3) are generally anti-inflammatory. A severe, chronic imbalance in these two types of eicosanoids will result in physical degeneration.

ESCHERICHIA COLI

Escherichia coli (commonly E. coli), is a bacterium that is commonly found in the lower intestine of warm-blooded animals. Most E. coli strains are harmless, but some, such as serotype O157:H7, can cause serious food poisoning in humans. The harmless strains are part of the normal flora of the gut, and can benefit their hosts by producing vitamin K_2, or by preventing the establishment of pathogenic bacteria within the intestine.

FATTY ACID

Fatty acids refers to the fats humans (and other animals) ingest as well as make within their bodies from unsaturated fatty acids ingested. Fatty acids are carbon chain acids, which may be saturated or unsaturated. Saturated acids are those whose carbon valances are all occupied with hydrogen. Unsaturated acids have unoccupied valances. Saturated acids may be burnt as fuel. The human (and other animals) body needs unsaturated acids for the construction and maintenance of its system.

FRUGIVOROUS

A frugivore is an animal that feeds primarily or, in some cases, exclusively on fruit. The diet of such animal is referred to as frugivorous.

HEMP SEED

Hemp seeds contain all the essential amino acids and essential fatty acids necessary to maintain healthy human life. 30–35% of the weight of hemp seed is oil containing 80% essential fatty acids (EFAs), linoleic acid (LA, 50-70%), alpha-linolenic acid (ALA, 15–25%) and gamma-linolenic acid (GLA, 1–6%). This is a good proportion for essential fatty acid consumption for human beings, and human health. In addition to oil, the seeds can be used to make hemp milk or hemp butter.

HYPERTENSION

Hypertension, also referred to as high blood pressure, HTN or HPN, is a medical condition in which the blood pressure is chronically elevated. In current usage, the word "hypertension" without a qualifier normally refers to arterial hypertension. Persistent hypertension is one of the risk factors for strokes, heart attacks, heart failure and arterial aneurysm, and is a leading cause of chronic renal failure. Even moderate elevation of arterial blood pressure leads to shortened life expectancy.

IMMUNOREGULATORY

Immunoregulatory refers to genes and other molecules, and processes, which control components of the immune system, such a T cells, such that they are deployed in proper numbers and do not act against 'self,' the body's own cells.

INFLAMMATION

Inflammation (Latin, inflamatio, to set on fire) is the complex biological response of vascular tissues to harmful stimuli, such as pathogens, damaged cells, or irritants. It is a protective attempt by the organism to remove the injurious stimuli as well as initiate the healing process for the tissue. In the absence of inflammation, wounds and infections would never heal and progressive destruction of the tissue would compromise the survival of the organism. However, inflammation which runs unchecked can also lead to a host of diseases, such as hay fever, atherosclerosis, and rheumatoid arthritis. It is for this reason that inflammation is normally tightly regulated by the body.

IRRADIATION

Irradiation refers to exposing foods (or medical implements, etc.) to an ionizing radiation for the purpose of killing pathogenic bacteria. Before 2000 foods were irradiated with radioactive cobalt. Since 2000 irradiation is done with high doses of electron beams. Foods subjected to such irradiation are free of harmful microorganisms; most of their nutrients have also been destroyed.

ISCHEMIC HEART DISEASE

Ischemic or ischaemic heart disease, or myocardial ischemia, is a disease characterized by a reduced flow of blood to the heart. It could be caused by atherosclerosis, high hypertension, or hypercholesterolemia. Depending on its severity, it could be treated orthomolecularly, pharmaceutically, by angioplasty, or coronary artery bypass surgery. It is the most common cause of death in the United States and most Western countries, and a major cause of hospital admissions.

JAKOB-CREUTZFELDT DISEASE

Creutzfeldt-Jakob disease (CJD) is a very rare and incurable degenerative neurological disorder (brain disease) that is ultimately fatal. Among the types of transmissible spongiform encephalopathy found in humans, it is the most common. It is considered to be a prion disease, a prion being a misshapen protein, which is reproduced in the body, and introduced into the brain. It is acquired by cannibalism, or by the eating of another animal which has transmissible spongiform encephalopathy.

LEGUMES

A legume is a plant in the family Fabaceae (or Leguminosae), or a fruit of these specific plants. A legume fruit is a simple dry fruit that develops from a simple carpel which usually opens along a seam on two sides. Well-known legumes include alfalfa, clover, peas, beans, lentils, mesquite, carob, and peanuts.

MRSA

MRSA is the acronym for Methicillin-Resistant Staphylococcus Aureus, and refers to the fact that such varieties of Staphylococcus have become resistant to antibiotics because of their overuse.

MYOCARDIAL INFARCTION

Myocardial infarction (MI or AMI for acute myocardial infarction), also known as a heart attack, occurs when the blood supply to part of the heart is interrupted. This is most commonly due to occlusion (blockage) of a coronary artery following the rupture of a vulnerable atherosclerotic plaque, which is an unstable collection of lipids (like cholesterol) and white blood cells (especially macrophages) in the wall of an artery. The resulting ischemia (restriction in blood supply) and oxygen shortage, if left untreated for a sufficient period, can cause damage and/or death (infarction) of heart muscle tissue (myocardium).

NEOLITHIC

Neolithic is a Greek term in Latin letters which means "new" "stone," and refers to the New Stone Age, the last of the periods in which human technology was fashioned by stone. The New Stone Age began at about 10,000 B.C.E. in the Middle East.

NEOPLASM

Neoplasia (new growth in Greek) is the abnormal proliferation of cells, resulting in a structure known as a neoplasm. The growth of this clone of cells exceeds, and is uncoordinated with, that of the normal tissues around it. It usually causes a lump or tumor. Neoplasms may be benign, pre-malignant or malignant. A malignant neoplasm is a cancer.

OMEGA 3 FATTY ACID

Omega 3 (n-3) fatty acid is one of the two essential fatty acids for the human body. Important nutritionally essential n-3 fatty acids are: alpha-linolenic acid (ALA), eicosapentaenoic acid (EPA), and docosahexaenoic acid (DHA). The human body cannot synthesize n-3 fatty acids de novo, but it can form 20- and 22-carbon unsaturated n-3 fatty acids from the eighteen-carbon n-3 fatty acid, alpha-linolenic acid.

OMEGA 6 FATTY ACID

Omega 6 (n-6) fatty acid is one of the two essential fatty acids for the human body. Important nutritionally essential n-6 fatty acids are: linoleic acid, and its derivatives: gamma-linolenic acid, arachidonic acid and others. The human body cannot synthesize n-6 fatty acid de novo, but it can form 20- and 22=carbon unsaturated n-6 fatty acids from the eighteen-carbon n-6 fatty acid, linoleic acid.

OSTEOPOROSIS

Osteoporosis is a disease of bone that leads to an increased risk of fracture. In osteoporosis the bone mineral density (BMD) is reduced, bone microarchitecture is disrupted, and the amount and variety of non-collagenous proteins in bone is altered. Osteoporosis is most common in women after menopause, when it is called postmenopausal osteoporosis, but may also develop in men, and may occur in anyone in the presence of particular hormonal disorders and other chronic diseases or as a result of medications, specifically glucocorticoids.

PALEOWATER

Paleowater is a synonym for fossil water, and refers to water which has been resident in an aquifer for a very long time, in the tens of thousands or millions of years.

PATHOGENIC

A pathogen is an infectious agent, referred to as a germ, which is a bacterium, a fungus, or a protist, which invades an animal body and disrupts it functioning. Most such invasions are by bacteria. The healthy human body has numerous defenses against many pathogenic bacteria, which can neutralize them. But, if a human is weakened by injury or by degeneration, many defenses may not be available, and such a human can more readily succumb to a bacterial infection or disease.

PH

PH, now usually expressed pH, is the measure of the acidity or alkalinity of a solution. It is a scale in which 7 is neutral. A pH lower than 7 is acidic. A pH higher than 7 is alkaline.

PHARMACEUTICAL

Pharmaceutical refers to the patented medicine method of treatment. It is currently the dominant method of medical treatment. In most cases treatment consists of administering a drug considered appropriate to the condition diagnosed. For non-pathogenic conditions, nutritive deficiency, or physical activity factors are not considered. A cure of the condition is usually not expected. This method of treatment is distinguished from orthomolecular treatment.

PHOSPHOLIPIDS Phospholipids are a class of lipids and are a major component of all biological membranes. This membrane is partially permeable, capable of elastic movement, and has fluid properties, in which embedded proteins (integral or peripheral proteins) and phospholipid molecules are able to move laterally.

PLAYA A playa is a dry or ephemeral lake bed. Playas are typically formed in semi-arid to arid regions of the world. The largest concentration of playa lakes in the world (nearly 22,000) is on the southern High Plains of Texas and eastern New Mexico.

POLYUNSATURATED FATTY ACID Polyunsaturated fatty acids (PUFA) are those which contain more than one double bond.

RESOLVINS Resolvins, Resolution-phase Interaction Products, are molecules derived from alpha-linolenic acid (omega 3) which are anti-inflammatory. Specifically, the derived acids, eicosapentaenoic acid and docosahexaenic acid, for Series E and Series D resolvins, respectively.

RUMINANT Physiologically, a ruminant is a mammal of the order Artiodactyla that digests plant-based food by initially softening it within the animal's first stomach, known as the rumen, then regurgitating the semi-digested mass, now known as cud, and chewing it again. The process of again chewing the cud to further break down plant matter and stimulate digestion is called "ruminating." Animals which ruminate include cattle, goats, sheep, antelope, and bisons.

SATURATED FATTY ACID	A saturated fatty acid is a carbon chain acid with all of the carbon valences occupied by hydrogen atoms. Foods that contain a high proportion of saturated fatty acids are cheese, butter, meats, coconut oil, and palm kernel oil.
SYMBIOTIC	Symbiotic is the adjective of symbiosis, which is the close and often long term interactions of different species. Usually there is mutual benefit for both or all of the interacting species. There is a symbiotic relationship between humans and their internal bacterial colonies.
THROMBOSIS	Thrombosis is the formation of a blood clot (thrombus) inside a blood vessel, obstructing the flow of blood through the circulatory system. When a blood vessel is injured, the body uses platelets and fibrin to form a blood clot, as the first step in repairing it (hemostasis) to prevent loss of blood. If that mechanism causes too much clotting, and the clot breaks free, a thrombus is formed.
TOXIN	A toxin is a poisonous substance produced by living cells or organisms that is active at very low concentrations. Toxins can be small molecules, peptides, or proteins and are capable of causing disease on contact or absorption with body tissues by interacting with biological macromolecules such as enzymes or cellular receptors. Toxins vary greatly in their severity, ranging from usually minor and acute (as in a bee sting) to almost immediately deadly (as in botulinum toxin).
TRIGLYCERIDE	Triglycerides are formed from a single molecule of glycerol, combined with three fatty acids, and make up most of fats digested by humans.

Ester bonds form between each fatty acid and the glycerol molecule. This is where the enzyme pancreatic lipase acts, hydrolyzing the bond and 'releasing' the fatty acid.

VADOSE ZONE

The vadose zone, also termed the unsaturated zone, is the portion of Earth between the land surface and the phreatic zone or zone of saturation ("vadose" is Latin for "shallow"). It extends from the top of the ground surface to the water table.

Index

www.ingramcontent.com/pod-product-compliance
Lightning Source LLC
Chambersburg PA
CBHW020436290526
45785CB00002B/881